WHAT TO EAT

DURING CANCER TREATMENT

More than 130 Recipes to Help You Cope

WHAT TO EAT

DURING CANCER TREATMENT

Jeanne Besser and Barbara L. Grant, MS, RDN, CSO
with the American Cancer Society

SECOND EDITION

American
Cancer
Society®

Published by the American Cancer Society

250 Williams Street NW, Atlanta, GA 30303-1002

Copyright ©2019 American Cancer Society

First edition 2009. Second edition 2019.

Printed in Canada

5 4 3 2 1   19 20 21 22 23

Recipes shown on cover, clockwise from top: Chickpea and Sweet Potato Curry, p. 243; Cranberry-Lime Granita, p. 148; Date and Fruit Bread, p. 109; Miso-Chicken Soup, p. 50. Back cover, clockwise from bottom: Raspberry Chia Pudding, p. 121; Rosemary Sweet and Spicy Nuts, p. 222; Carrot-Ginger Drink, p. 34; Lemon-Herb Tilapia Packets, p. 76.

Additional Photo Credits: p. 6, Tatiana Bralnina/shutterstock.com; p. 9, baibaz/shutterstock.com; p. 10, Brooke Becker/shutterstock.com; p. 11, Africa Studio/shutterstock.com; p. 17 (top to bottom), Lana Langlois/shutterstock.com, Hong Vo/shutterstock.com; p. 18, eugena-klykova/shutterstock.com; p.19, Andrei Kuzmik/shutterstock.com; p.21, squarelogo/shutterstock.com; p. 248, Foxys Forest Manufacture/shutterstock.com; p. 255 (top to bottom), Dan Thornberg/shutterstock.com, AG-PHOTOS/shutterstock.com, Sashkin/shutterstock.com, Lipskiy/shutterstock.com, Tatiana Popova/shutterstock.com, Africa Studio/shutterstock.com

Library of Congress Cataloging-in-Publication Data is available.

Photography by Angie Mosier

Food styling by Jeanne Besser

Design and composition by Katie Jennings Campbell

Indexing by Bob Land

Nutritional analysis by Madelyn Wheeler, MS, RD

American Cancer Society

Editorial and Production

Senior Vice President, Cancer Control Programs and Services: Chuck Westbrook

Managing Director, Content: Eleni Berger

Senior Director, Journals and Book Publishing: Esmeralda Galán Buchanan

Book Publishing Manager: Vanika Jordan, MSPub

Senior Editor, Book Publishing: Jill Russell

Medical and Nutritional Review

Managing Director, Nutrition and Physical Activity: Colleen Doyle, MS, RD

Director, Cancer Information: Amy Sherrod, RN, MSN, CPNP

Medical Editor: Mamta Kalidas, MD

Associate Editor: Mahal Lynn Gadd, MSN, MBA, RN, OCN

Quantity discounts on bulk purchases of this book are available. For information, please send an e-mail to trade.sales@cancer.org. For general inquiries about American Cancer Society books, send an e-mail to acsbooks@cancer.org.

For more information about cancer, contact your American Cancer Society at 800-227-2345 or cancer.org.

CONTENTS

NAUSEA N

DIARRHEA D

CONSTIPATION `C`

TROUBLE SWALLOWING TS

SORE MOUTH OR THROAT SM

UNINTENTIONAL WEIGHT LOSS WL

TASTE CHANGES `TC`

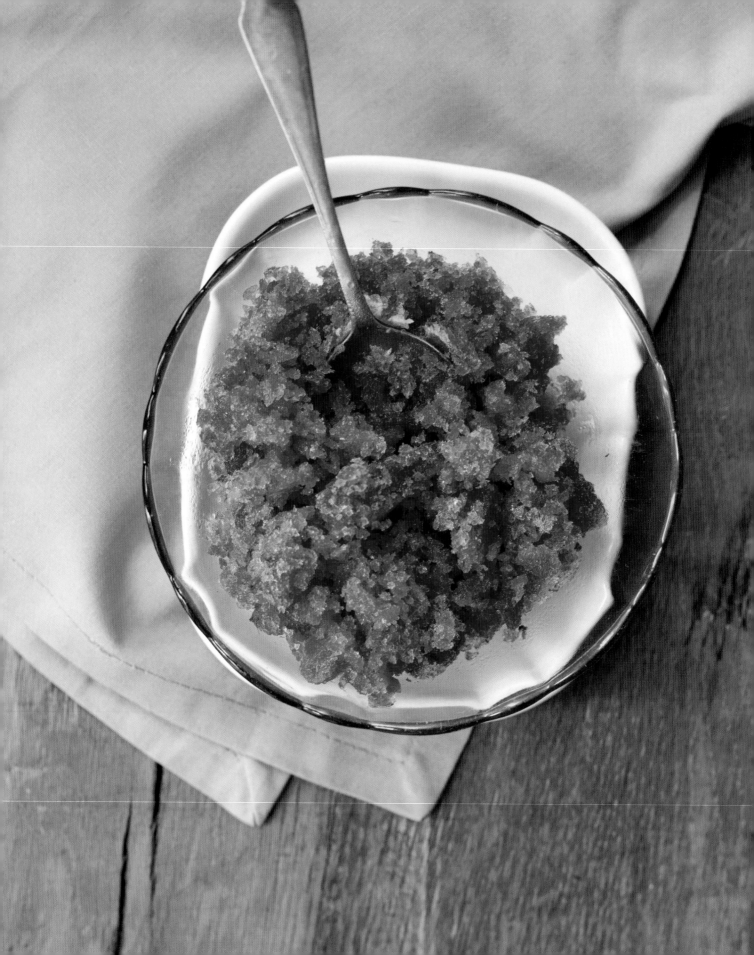

INTRODUCTION

If you are reading this, you or someone you know is going through or preparing for cancer treatment. A cancer diagnosis is life changing, and this can be a stressful and difficult time, a time often filled with challenges and change. Not everyone experiences side effects, and for those who do, not everyone experiences the same side effects or experiences them in the same way. A person going through cancer treatment has unique nutritional needs and issues related to eating; what's more, these needs may change throughout the cancer experience. Your appetite may change from day to day. Foods may not taste or smell the way they did before treatment, and you may be surprised by some of the foods that appeal to you. You may have to deal with unintended weight loss or gain.

Many people going through cancer ask if diet and nutrition can help them fight and recover from cancer. The answer is yes! No matter what side effects you experience, nutrition will be an essential part of dealing with your cancer and cancer treatment. Healthy eating and staying hydrated can help fuel recovery, help you manage side effects, and keep your body strong.

Some people going through cancer treatment continue to enjoy eating and have a normal appetite throughout treatment. Others have days when they don't feel like eating at all. For many, side effects come and go. Not eating enough can lead to weight loss, and weight loss can lead to weakness and fatigue. Eating as well as you can during your treatment and your recovery is an important part of taking care of yourself.

There are no hard and fast rules about how to eat during cancer treatment. Eat as healthfully as possible—the importance of this cannot be overstated. However, eating during treatment may be different in many ways from how you ate before. Eating well does not mean that you need to be perfect. Try to select a variety of nutritious foods each day to help keep your body healthy. But do not be too hard on yourself if the foods you can tolerate are not the most nutritious or if you have days during which your appetite is poor. There will be times when what you can eat is impacted by your treatment and its effect on your body.

You will find some recipes in this book that are higher in calories, fat, or sugar than typically recommended as part of the daily diet for someone without cancer. Managing side effects can require a different approach. Balance is key, and the nutritional needs of a person going through cancer treatment are unique and different from those of someone without cancer.

In many ways, this is not a typical cookbook. Recipes are organized by side effect: nausea, diarrhea, constipation, trouble swallowing, sore mouth or throat, unintentional weight loss, and taste changes. As you're reading through the recipes, look for these symbols at the top of the page:

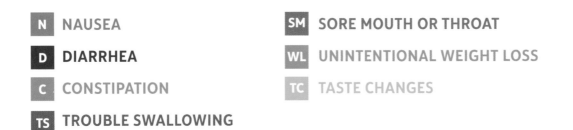

For reference, a couple of lists are included to help you find the recipes that will be most useful to you. In the beginning of the book, there is a list of all recipes by chapter, with symbols beside each indicating the side effects for which it is appropriate. At the back of the book (pages 261–266), you will also find a complete list of recipes for each side effect, to give a clear, easy-to-understand picture of what might be best for you. Keep in mind that many of the recipes work for people dealing with more than one side effect. For example, the Raspberry Chia Pudding on page 121 appears in the chapter for constipation, but may also be appropriate if you are experiencing taste changes, so both the C and TC icons appear on that page.

Most people with cancer have families that are going through this experience along with them. While the recipes are focused on a cancer patient's specific needs, most are also nutritious and easy to prepare and are also intended for the family or caretaker to enjoy. Since these recipes are written for people who are undergoing treatment, some are mildly flavored. Tips throughout the book give suggestions for ways to adapt the recipes for family members or for when the side effect has resolved. As you start to feel better, you can tweak the recipes to suit your changing tastes and needs.

Some people with cancer are also dealing with other health problems, such as diabetes, heart disease, or high blood pressure. Many of the recipes in this book are appropriate for people with other health issues, but if this applies to you, make sure your regular doctors know you are being treated for cancer, and always follow the advice of your health care team. If you are already on a diet for a particular health condition, make sure that you speak with your doctor before you make changes.

This second edition also comes with updated and expanded content that will be of great use to anyone going through cancer treatment. This information is based on years of experience working with patients and helping them navigate that process. On pages 8-9, advice is given for the caregiver. Taking care of someone who is going through cancer treatment can be challenging, but also rewarding. On pages 10-16, guidance is provided on food safety for someone going through treatment. Food safety is very important during treatment, when your immune system can be compromised and more vulnerable to foodborne infections. On pages 17-19, you'll find information on snacking and staying hydrated. A section addressing some common questions is on pages 20-22. Vitamin and mineral deficiencies during treatment are discussed on pages 23-25. See page 26 for information about how to deal with weight gain during treatment. While less common than weight loss, it is still a problem that affects many people. And new to this edition, a section has been added on eating and living well after treatment (pages 249-258).

During active cancer treatment, your overall nutritional goal should be to eat a variety of foods that provide the nutrients needed to maintain health while you fight cancer. Try to do these things every day, when possible:

- Eat regular meals and snacks throughout the day.

- Include an array of colorful fruits and vegetables in your diet.

- Incorporate good sources of protein in your diet, including plant-based proteins such as nuts, seeds, beans, and peas.

- Drink plenty of water and other hydrating fluids.

- As you are able, be physically active, and try to avoid inactivity.

- Strive to obtain and maintain a healthy weight during treatment, with your doctor's guidance.

- Keep your cupboards and refrigerator stocked with foods and snacks so that you have ready-to-eat items on hand for times when you are not feeling well.

- Plan ahead by cooking in advance and freezing foods in meal-sized portions.

- Do not be afraid to try new foods, especially if favorite foods are tasting different or unpleasant.

Most cancer centers have a registered dietitian (RD) on staff to help patients. Talk with your health care team about any nutrition- and diet-related concerns you have and ask them for a referral. Working one-on-one with the RD can help you create an individualized plan for your situation. If one is not available at your clinic or medical center, contact the American Cancer Society at 800-227-2345, or you can also go to the Academy of Nutrition and Dietetics website at eatright.org/find-an-expert to locate an RD who specializes in oncology nutrition in your area.

Whether you need help dealing with side effects or simply want to make sure you maintain your health, this cookbook was written to help you. These recipes and suggestions were written to make this time a little bit easier for everyone. Every person is different, and your cancer experience will be unique. As mentioned earlier, there are no hard and fast rules about how to eat during cancer treatment. With experimentation, you can learn what works best for you.

For more information about cancer, nutrition, and managing the side effects of treatment, contact the American Cancer Society at 800-227-2345 or cancer.org.

A FEW NOTES ABOUT THE RECIPES

As you read through recipes, pay particular attention to the introductory text and the tips—they contain helpful information about recipe preparation, ways to alter the recipes, and notes about conditions such as low white blood cell counts (neutropenia).

Most recipes call for full-fat or "regular" dairy products instead of reduced-fat or nonfat items. Feel free to use a reduced-fat or nonfat option if that is more appropriate for your needs or appetite.

Each recipe includes full nutritional information for one serving. Serving sizes are approximate—exact serving sizes will depend on the size of your ingredients (vegetables, for example) and your preparation. When you are feeling unwell, just try to eat what you can. Keep these things in mind:

- Optional ingredients and ingredients listed without a specified amount ("Salt and freshly ground black pepper," for example) are not represented in the analysis, nor are ingredients suggested as possible accompaniments.

- When a recipe gives a choice of ingredients, the first option was used in the analysis.

- All data are rounded according to the U.S. Food and Drug Administration Rounding Rules.

- If a serving range is given, the analysis is for the smaller number of servings.

The information in this book is not official policy of the American Cancer Society and is not intended as medical advice to replace the expertise of your health care team. It is intended to help you and your family make informed decisions, together with your doctors.

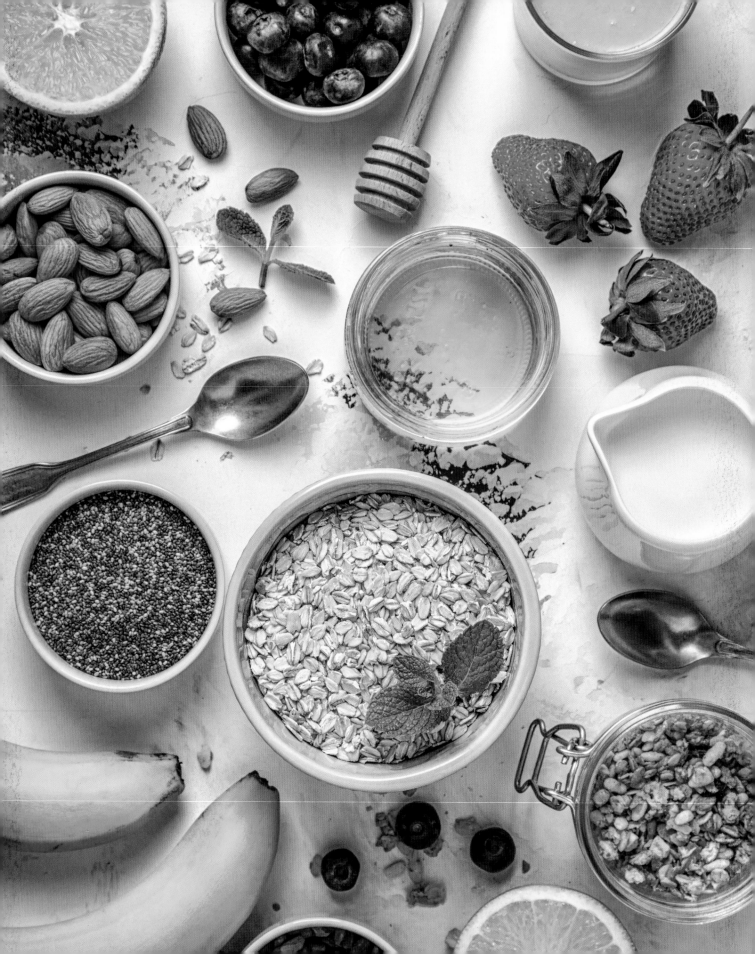

WHAT YOU NEED TO KNOW

ADVICE FOR THE CAREGIVER

If you are the caregiver, it can be frustrating and difficult at times to meet the nutritional needs of a person who may not feel like eating or whose likes and dislikes can change daily. Foods may not taste normal to someone going through cancer treatment, so don't be offended if old favorites aren't appealing. If the person's tastes seem to have changed, encourage new foods.

Don't worry if there are days when the person's diet is not as balanced as you would like. Sometimes the foods your loved one asks for or tolerates best may not be things you would normally consider to be part of a "healthy" diet. Of course, it is important to eat as well as possible during treatment, but there may be times when the goal is to take in as many calories as possible, or times when simply eating is a victory. Remember that it is okay for nutritional goals to be different right now, and days when the person is feeling better will make up for more challenging days.

Try to be patient and encouraging when your loved one does not feel like eating, and look for opportunities to make eating easier. Keep the fridge, freezer, and pantry stocked with easy-to-prepare foods and things that can be eaten as is. Many people going through cancer treatment experience lack of appetite or other problems that can make eating daunting or difficult. A large plate of food can be overwhelming. It sometimes works better for patients dealing with side effects to snack or eat small meals throughout the day, instead of three large meals. See page 18 for ideas for easy snacks to keep on hand or include in a basket or cooler near the couch or a favorite chair. Keeping snacks nearby can make it easier for your loved one to nibble when they do feel like eating. Also, keep items that he or she normally eats and tolerates well when sick.

Here are some other tips that you may find helpful:

- Try to make mealtimes pleasant, as much as possible. Play music, watch a movie, or have friends over if he or she is up to it.

- Offer the biggest meal of the day when he or she feels the hungriest—for many people, this is in the morning.

- Offer favorite foods any time of the day. It's okay to have a sandwich or bowl of soup for breakfast or have breakfast food for dinner.

- Package leftovers in single-serving containers for future meals; large servings can seem overwhelming when someone's appetite is poor.

■ If your loved one is sensitive to smells, prepare meals in a different room from where they'll be eaten. Suggest that he or she go to another room while food is being prepared. If possible, consider grilling outdoors or using a slow cooker on the back porch or in the garage to keep the smell of food from filling the house. Serving foods cool or at room temperature also decreases aromas.

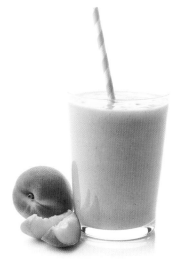

■ Drinking is often easier than eating. If your loved one does not feel like eating but is willing to drink, offer sips of smoothies, soups, nutritional supplements, hot cocoa, milk, and milk shakes. Soups can be sipped out of mugs and reheated as needed. Cups with lids will also help block smells.

It is always important to follow food safety procedures, but it is especially important if you are preparing meals for someone undergoing cancer treatment, as it may reduce the person's ability to fight off infections. The next section provides an overview of keeping food safe for everyone; familiarize yourself with these basics and be sure to put them into practice.

Most importantly, remember that you cannot do it all yourself. Caregiving can be demanding, and it is not realistic or healthy to try to tackle everything on your own. When friends or family offer to help, accept, even if it is difficult. Look for situations where you need assistance, and jot ideas down in a notepad or on your phone. There are many ways people can help: meals, grocery shopping, helping with yardwork or housecleaning, babysitting, or even just staying with your loved one so that you can take a break. Ask others what they can do to give you a hand, and be clear about what you need. People want to help but often struggle with knowing how best to provide the assistance you need. Remember how important it is that you also take care of yourself during this time! Eating well, being as active as possible, getting enough sleep, and practicing stress-reduction techniques can help you stay at your best so that you can offer the best care.

FOOD SAFETY DURING CANCER TREATMENT

There may be times during cancer treatment when the body is not able to protect itself very well. Cancer and its treatment can weaken the body's immune system by affecting the blood cells that protect against germs. When your immune system is weakened, the first step in staying free from infection is being aware of and avoiding the bacteria and other organisms that can make you ill. Following safe food practices can reduce the risk of foodborne illness. Follow the practices outlined in this section to maintain good food safety.

Some foods should be avoided by anyone going through cancer treatment. These foods can contain high levels of bacteria:

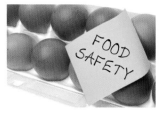

- Undercooked meat or poultry, especially ground meats

- Raw or runny eggs, including nonpasteurized or homemade eggnog, smoothies or drinks made with raw eggs, unbaked meringues, or Caesar salad dressing made with raw egg

- Nonpasteurized vegetable and fruit juice, unless prepared at home with washed produce

- Uncooked vegetable sprouts (all kinds, including alfalfa, radish, broccoli, mung bean, etc.), because of a high risk of contamination with salmonella and E. coli

CLEANING PROPERLY

- Wash your hands with warm, soapy water for twenty seconds before and after preparing food and after using the bathroom or touching pets. Always wash hands before eating.

- Clean counters and cutting boards with hot, soapy water or a fresh solution made of one part bleach to ten parts water. Moist disinfecting wipes may be used if they're made for use around food.

- Use paper towels to clean kitchen surfaces. Cloth kitchen towels should be replaced daily and laundered in hot water.

WHAT IS NEUTROPENIA?

Some types of cancer treatment can cause a condition known as neutropenia, or low white blood cell counts. Having neutropenia puts one at greater risk for infection and foodborne illnesses. If this happens, ask your health care team if you should follow specific diet guidelines. When white blood cell counts are low, your health care team may tell you to avoid additional foods.

- Wash fruits and vegetables well under running water before peeling or cutting. Do not use soaps, detergents, or chlorine bleach solutions. With a clean vegetable scrubber, scrub produce that has a thick and rough skin or rind (such as melons, potatoes, bananas, etc.) or any produce that has dirt on it.

- Packaged salads, slaw mixes, and other prepared produce, even when marked prewashed, should be rinsed again under running water. Using a colander or salad spinner can make this easier.

- Wash the tops of canned goods with soap and water before opening.

HEATING AND STORING FOOD

- Keep hot foods hot (warmer than 140°F) and cold foods cold (cooler than 40°F).

- Keep your refrigerator set at or below 40°F. Use an appliance thermometer to be sure.

- Do not refreeze foods once you've thawed them.

- Refrigerate meat, poultry, seafood, eggs, and other perishable foods within two hours of buying or preparing them. Egg dishes and cream- and mayonnaise-based foods should not be left unrefrigerated.

- If preparing hot food that won't be served right away (or that you'll be freezing or transporting later), divide into shallow dishes or containers so that it cools more quickly in the refrigerator.

- Throw away fruits and vegetables that are slimy or moldy.

- Throw away eggs with cracked shells.

- Throw out foods that look or smell strange. Never taste them!

- Discard food that has not been eaten in an appropriate timeframe. See the guidance on the next page for how long to keep specific foods on hand.

AVOIDING CROSS-CONTAMINATION

- Keep raw meat, poultry, or seafood separated from other foods, both when grocery shopping and in the refrigerator.

- If thawing raw meat or poultry in the refrigerator, place in a container to catch liquid. If possible, place the thawing food on a lower shelf in the refrigerator.

- Keep foods separated on the countertops. Use separate cutting boards and clean knives for raw meats and other foods.

- When grilling, always use a clean plate for the cooked meat.

- Marinades used on raw food should not be used as a sauce. Reserve a portion before putting raw meat or poultry in it.

COOKING FOOD WELL

- Ensure all meats, poultry, and fish are cooked thoroughly. Use a food thermometer placed into the thickest part of the food to be sure that meat and poultry reach the proper temperature. (See the chart of safe food temperatures on page 16.) Test a thermometer's accuracy by putting it into boiling water—it should read 212°F.

- When cooking in the microwave, rotate the dish a quarter turn once or twice during cooking if there's no turntable in the oven. This helps prevent cold spots in food where bacteria can survive.

- Cover leftovers when reheating. All leftovers should be brought to a minimum temperature of 165 degrees.

- Cook eggs until both whites and yolks are firm, not runny.

- When reheating soups, sauces, or gravies, be sure to bring to a boil.

COLD FOOD STORAGE

When storing food in your refrigerator, follow these food storage safety guidelines.

FOOD	STORAGE TIME (40°F)
Eggs	
Eggs (fresh)	3 to 5 weeks
Eggs (hard-boiled)	1 week
Liquid pasteurized eggs, egg substitutes (opened)	3 days
Liquid pasteurized eggs, egg substitutes (unopened)	10 days
Poultry, Seafood, and Fresh Meats	
Fresh poultry	1 to 2 days
Seafood	1 to 2 days
Fresh beef, veal, lamb, pork*	3 to 5 days
Hamburger and other ground meats*	1 to 2 days
Prepared Foods and Lunch Meats	
Egg, chicken, ham, tuna, and macaroni salads*	3 to 5 days
Lunch meat (open)*	3 to 5 days
Lunch meat (unopened)*	2 weeks
Hot dogs (open)*	1 week
Hot dogs (unopened)*	2 weeks
Bacon*	7 days
Sausage, raw*	1 to 2 days
Leftovers	3 to 4 days

Because of their link to increased cancer risk, the American Cancer Society recommends limiting consumption of red and processed meat. However, if you are consuming these foods, follow the guidance above for safe storage.

CHOOSING FOOD CAREFULLY

- Check "sell-by" and "use-by" dates. Pick only the freshest products.

- Check the packaging date on fresh meats, poultry, and seafood. Do not buy products that are out of date.

- Do not use damaged, swollen, rusted, or deeply dented cans. Be sure that packaged and boxed foods are properly sealed.

- Choose unblemished fruits and vegetables.

- Do not buy produce that has been cut at the grocery store (such as melon or sliced onions).

- Do not eat deli foods prepared at the grocery store. In the bakery, avoid unrefrigerated cream- and custard-filled desserts and pastries.

- Do not eat foods from self-serve or bulk containers unless they will be cooked.

- Do not eat yogurt and ice cream products from soft-serve machines.

- Do not eat food samples.

- Only purchase refrigerated eggs, and check to be sure there are no cracked eggs.

- Choose salsas or salad dressings that are shelf-stable, not items in the refrigerated section of the store.

- Put meats, poultry, and seafood in plastic bags and put them in a separate area of the cart. At the check-out, ask that they be bagged separately from other food items.

- Get your frozen and refrigerated foods just before you check out, especially during summer months.

- Never leave food in a hot car. Refrigerate groceries right away. If you live far from the grocery store or it is very hot, take a cooler or thermal bags for frozen and refrigerated items.

EATING OUT SAFELY

- Try to dine early to avoid crowds.

- In fast-food restaurants, ask that food be prepared fresh. Ask for a modification from how it's normally prepared (without onions, for example) to ensure your food is made to order.

- Ask for single-serving condiment packages, and avoid self-serve bulk condiment containers.

- Avoid salad bars, delicatessens, buffets and smorgasbords, potlucks, sidewalk vendors, and food trucks.

- Avoid "fresh-squeezed" juices or sliced lemons or limes in restaurants or other food service establishments.

- Be sure that utensils are put on a napkin or clean tablecloth or placemat, rather than right on the table.

- If you want to keep your leftovers, ask for a container and put the food in it yourself rather than having the server take your food to the kitchen to do this.

- Refrigerate leftovers as soon as possible, definitely within two hours. If the temperature outside is above 90 degrees, refrigerate them within an hour.

TAKING FOOD TO FRIENDS

One easy way to help someone going through treatment is to prepare food for his or her family. There are several online meal-organizing platforms now available that allow people to coordinate to provide meals for others. There are a few things that can be useful to remember in this situation:

- Don't send food in a container you need back. Avoid a situation in which the family has to be responsible for washing a dish, remembering whom it belonged to, and arranging to return it. Send food in disposable containers or include a note saying the dish doesn't need to be returned.

- Pay careful attention to these food safety guidelines, particularly with regards to transporting food and maintaining safe food temperatures.

- Consider asking whether the person would like anything specific or has any current favorites. Don't try to impress—comfort food is usually most desired.

- Touch base if possible to be sure there aren't food allergies or special dietary needs. Especially during treatment, a person's tastes may change, or there may be certain foods that are particularly easy or difficult to tolerate. If you bring something homemade, consider providing a list of ingredients.

- On sign-ins, give an idea of what you are bringing (or send an e-mail to check) so that the same foods aren't repeated.

Remember that even if the person with cancer can't eat everything you bring, the family will enjoy it. Your effort will be appreciated, and you are helping to ease a burden.

MINIMUM INTERNAL COOKING TEMPERATURES

You can't tell if certain foods are safe to eat just by looking. Use a food thermometer to be sure. Use the following guidelines for safe internal cooking temperatures.

FOOD	COOKING TEMPERATURE
Eggs, Egg Dishes, and Casseroles	
Eggs	Cook until yolk and white are firm
Egg dishes, custards	160°F
Seafood	
Fish (such as salmon, cod, halibut, snapper, sole, bass, trout)	145°F or cook until opaque and flesh flakes easily with a fork
Shrimp, lobster, crab	Cook until flesh is pearly opaque
Scallops	Should turn milky white or opaque and firm
Clams, mussels, oysters	Cook until shells open (may be high-risk for people with low white blood cell count or immunosuppression)
Poultry (Chicken, Turkey, Duck, Goose)	
Chicken and turkey: whole bird	165°F
Breast, roast	165°F
Ground chicken, turkey	165°F
Stuffing (cook in separate container outside of bird)	165°F
Veal, Beef, Pork, Lamb, Rabbit, Goat, Game*	
Whole pieces of meat, hot dogs*	145°F
Ground veal, beef, lamb, pork, rabbit, goat, game*	160°F
Ham	
Fresh (raw)*	145°F
Precooked (to reheat)*	140°F
Leftovers	
Leftovers and casseroles	165°F

*Because of their link to increased cancer risk, the American Cancer Society recommends limiting consumption of red and processed meat. However, if you are consuming these foods, follow the guidance above for safe cooking temperature.

SNACKING, STAYING HYDRATED, AND THE "SURVIVAL KIT"

Good nutrition, adequate calorie intake, and staying hydrated can help maintain energy, stamina, and strength during your treatment. However, many types of treatment can affect your appetite and desire to eat and drink. When you do feel hungry, for example, the feeling may not last long, so it is important to take advantage of it when it does appear.

Consider making a "survival kit" to keep handy next to your favorite chair or spot on the couch so that foods and beverages are easily accessible. An insulated lunch box or small cooler with some quick and easy snacks and drinks is an easy way to capitalize on moments when you want to eat, helping you maintain your weight and hydration when your appetite is poor. Single-serving snacks and resealable packaging are helpful.

Here are some suggestions for your cooler:

- Make sure to have beverages on hand, such as bottled water, juice boxes, and sports drinks. Packaged nutritional supplements can help during times you feel like drinking but not eating.

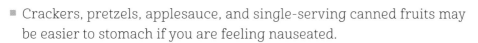

- Use an ice pack to keep cold foods such as yogurt, individually wrapped cheeses, cottage cheese, hard-boiled eggs, gelatin, and puddings chilled throughout the day.

- Crackers, pretzels, applesauce, and single-serving canned fruits may be easier to stomach if you are feeling nauseated.

- Dips with beans or cheese can add variety and protein to your snacks.

- Keep a mixture of sweet and salty snacks on hand to satisfy any cravings.

- For high-calorie snacks that don't require any preparation, try canned fruit in syrup, peanut butter and crackers, dried fruit, nuts, cheese and crackers, trail mix, granola, and energy bars.

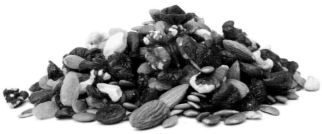

EASY SNACKS TO KEEP ON HAND DURING TREATMENT

Instant breakfast drinks

Applesauce

Gelatin

Puddings

Cereals (cold and warm)

Crackers, pretzels, and rice cakes

Nuts and seeds

Peanut butter and other nut butters

Pita bread and hummus

Hard-boiled eggs

Apple slices, bananas, orange sections, or other fresh fruit

Canned fruit

Dried fruit, fruit leather

Frozen grapes and cherries

Granola and granola bars, protein bars, energy bars

Popcorn

Trail mix

Yogurt

Cheese

Sorbet

Popsicles

Sherbet

Frozen yogurt

Ice cream

Carrot and celery sticks

Tortillas, quesadillas

Refried beans, dips made with beans

Bagels and cream cheese

Muffins

Staying Hydrated

Good hydration is important to good health in general and is even more essential during cancer treatment. If you are having side effects such as vomiting or diarrhea, you will need to take in even more fluid. Staying hydrated can be a struggle, however, and you may grow weary of drinking water. Fortunately, there are many ways to get much-needed fluids into the body.

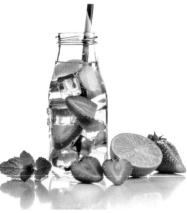

- Water (plain, with fruit, flavored, sparkling)

- Bouillon, broth, or consommé

- Pasteurized fruit and vegetable juices and nectars

- Fruit punch and other fruit-flavored drinks

- Sports drinks

- Caffeine-free hot or iced tea

- Gelatin (regular or sugar-free)

- Popsicles and flavored ice pops, fruit ices

- Coconut water

- Smoothies, milk shakes

- Milk, almond milk, soy milk

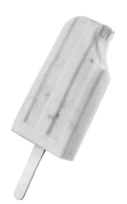

By the time you feel thirsty, your body most likely has already lost precious fluid, and you'll need to drink even more fluid to replace what's been lost. Try to keep a glass or bottle of water or another healthy fluid with you at all times so that you can sip throughout the day. Some people find it helpful to set a daily goal for a certain number of bottles or glasses of water or to keep a log of each glass or bottle consumed.

ANSWERS TO COMMON QUESTIONS

CAN I TAKE DIETARY SUPPLEMENTS DURING TREATMENT?

Dietary supplements include things like vitamins, minerals, herbs, and digestive enzymes. No matter what kind of cancer treatment you are getting, it's always best to talk with your doctor before starting any type of dietary supplement. If you have been taking supplements and want to keep taking them, it's important that your doctor knows this, too.

Many people assume that dietary supplements are always safe to take along with prescription medicine. This may not be true. Some vitamins and other dietary supplements can interfere with cancer treatments and medication or can even make treatment-related side effects worse.

Dietary supplements are also not regulated by the Food and Drug Administration or any other agency. Some dietary supplements are formulated under careful conditions in clean, controlled laboratories and labeled accurately. Others may contain some or none of the substances listed on their labels. And many supplements contain other substances that are not listed on their labels—fillers, different herbs, or actual drugs that are known to be able to cause harm. Others may be marketed as containing proprietary ingredients, and the amount of each item listed on the label is unknown.

Remember, too, that safety and dose are related. For many plants, such as culinary herbs used in cooking, the leaves or roots can be safely taken in small amounts. But concentrated extracts sold as liquids or pills may contain the plant's chemicals in far greater amounts and may not be safe.

Just because something is "all natural" does not necessarily mean it is safe. Keep in mind that some of the most toxic substances in the world occur naturally. Poisonous mushrooms, for example, are completely natural but not safe or helpful to humans.

Again, regardless of what type of treatment you're on, talk with your health care team about any supplements you are taking or wish to take.

DOES SUGAR FEED CANCER? SHOULD I ELIMINATE SUGAR FROM MY DIET?

Many people with cancer are concerned about sugar in their diets, often reacting to stories that sugar "feeds" cancer. This is a very common belief. All cells, including cancer cells, need glucose (blood sugar) for energy. But giving more sugar to cancer cells does not make them grow faster, and starving them of sugar does not make them grow more slowly.

The bigger problem is that too much sugar can contribute to weight gain, excess body fat, and obesity, which does increase cancer risk. Added sugars are typically found in foods that don't have any nutritional value, like sweetened drinks, cookies and cakes, and other highly processed foods. Sugar is low in nutrients and contributes little to the diet except calories, which can lead to unhealthy weight gain. Foods high in refined sugars and carbohydrates may also increase insulin resistance, which has been linked to diabetes, heart disease, and obesity. There is a clear link between obesity and increased cancer risk.

Not all sugar is bad—natural sugars found in such foods as fruit play an important part in a healthy diet. Other healthful foods containing natural sugars are vegetables, whole grains, and low-fat dairy foods. As part of a healthy diet, the American Heart Association recommends that women consume no more than six teaspoons (twenty-four grams) of sugar a day, and that men take in a maximum of nine teaspoons (thirty-six grams) per day.

But should you make efforts to avoid all sugar during treatment? The answer is no. During cancer treatment, there may be times when the priority is to get calories or stay hydrated, and how that happens is less important. Try to use sugar-containing foods and beverages sparingly during these times, and when you are feeling and eating better, make an effort to make healthful food choices. Talk with your health care team and registered dietitian to help you determine what foods are best for your situation. After treatment, a healthy diet is an important part of taking care of yourself. See pages 249–258 for more information on eating well after cancer treatment.

SHOULD I EAT ORGANIC FOODS?

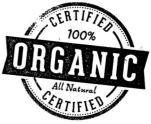

Organic food is different from conventionally produced food in the way it is grown, handled, and processed. The term "organic" is often used to refer to plant foods grown without pesticides and genetic modifications. It also refers to meat, poultry, eggs, and dairy products produced without antibiotics or growth hormones. Organic farming does not use bioengineering, ionizing radiation, conventional pesticides, or fertilizers made with synthetic ingredients or sewage sludge.

Organic foods contain fewer contaminants than conventionally produced foods. However, the United States Department of Agriculture (USDA) makes no claims that organically produced food is safer or more nutritious than conventionally produced food. Organic produce, like any produce, should be washed before eating. It may be organic, but it still could be contaminated by dirt, insects, or even stray pesticide residues.

It's important to remember that the term "natural" does not mean "organic." Food labeled as organic has been certified as meeting USDA organic standards. The term "natural" is not defined by law or in Food and Drug Administration regulations, so there are no guidelines or restrictions governing its use.

Several studies have looked at the nutrient content of organic versus conventionally grown fruits and vegetables, and while some studies suggest a higher nutrient content, others suggest no difference. It is possible that differences in nutrient content relate to the fact that organic foods are consumed earlier after harvest than are nonorganic foods, simply because the quality of organics can reduce rapidly. Generally, the closer produce is to the time of harvest, the higher the nutrient content, regardless of whether it is organic.

During cancer treatment, some people choose to eat organic foods to reduce exposure to pesticides. This is certainly an acceptable approach, but it may or may not change health, and it will likely increase food costs. The bottom line is this: if consuming mostly organic foods provides you with greater peace of mind, do it.

VITAMIN AND MINERAL DEFICIENCIES DURING TREATMENT

The body needs small amounts of vitamins and minerals to help it function properly, and a person who eats a balanced diet usually gets plenty of vitamins and minerals. But it can be hard to eat a balanced diet when you're being treated for cancer, especially if you have side effects that last a long time. In this case, your doctor or registered dietitian may suggest a daily multivitamin and mineral supplement. If you are struggling with eating for weeks or months, it's important your doctor know, as you might need to be checked for vitamin or mineral deficiencies.

Always talk with your doctor first if you're thinking of taking a vitamin or supplement. Some people with cancer take large amounts of vitamins, minerals, and other dietary supplements to try to boost their immune system or even destroy cancer cells. But some of these substances can be harmful, especially when taken in large doses. In fact, large doses of some vitamins and minerals may make some chemotherapy and radiation therapy regimens less effective or could possibly make side effects worse. See page 20 for more on dietary supplements.

Three of the most common deficiencies that occur during cancer treatment are deficiencies in iron, potassium, and magnesium. In addition to supplements or other treatments your doctor may prescribe, your registered dietitian may tell you to eat foods that are rich in these nutrients.

IRON DEFICIENCY ANEMIA

Iron deficiency anemia is the most common type of anemia and has been estimated to affect approximately 40 percent of cancer patients. It is a recognized side effect of certain types of chemotherapy, and many people who aren't anemic when their cancer is diagnosed will become anemic during treatment.

Iron deficiency anemia happens when the body is low in iron and cannot make hemoglobin—the part of the red blood cell that carries oxygen to all cells in the body. If your anemia becomes serious, you may need a blood transfusion or special medications. Your health care team will monitor your condition to determine whether additional care is needed.

If your anemia is mild, you may be asked to eat more iron-rich foods. Iron in food comes from two sources: animals and plants. Iron from animal sources, known as heme iron, is better absorbed by the body than iron from plant sources, known as nonheme iron.

GOOD SOURCES OF IRON

Chicken liver	Eggs	Lentils
Oysters	Shrimp	Molasses
Clams	Leg of lamb	Spinach
Beef liver	Cereals that are iron-enriched, such as Raisin Bran	Whole wheat bread
Beef (chuck roast, lean ground beef)	Instant oatmeal	Peanut butter
Turkey leg	Beans (kidney, lima, navy)	Brown rice
Tuna	Tofu	

Here are some ways to help your body increase iron absorption:

- Combine iron-containing foods or supplements with foods rich in vitamin C, such as oranges and other citrus fruits, tomatoes, broccoli, and strawberries.

- Eat both animal and plant sources of iron.

- Cook food in cast iron pans.

- If your health care provider prescribes an iron supplement, ask if you should take two or three small doses instead of one larger dose. The amount of iron your body can absorb at one time decreases as the dose increases.

The following things can make it harder for your body to absorb iron:

- Drinking large amounts of coffee or tea with foods that are high in iron

- Having more than 30 grams of fiber a day

- Eating foods high in calcium (such as dairy products or calcium-fortified juices) at the same time as foods high in iron

MAGNESIUM DEFICIENCY

Magnesium is a mineral important to the way our muscles and nerves function. It also helps keep your blood pressure at normal levels and improves bone strength. Some types of cancer treatment can cause magnesium levels to get low, and your doctor may tell you to eat a magnesium-rich diet as one way to help with this problem. A magnesium-rich diet is one that includes at least 400 milligrams of magnesium daily.

GOOD SOURCES OF MAGNESIUM

Dark green vegetables	Pumpkin seeds	Potato, baked with skin
Whole grains	Soy milk	Bran flakes
Bananas	Black beans	Oatmeal
Almonds	Spinach	Shredded wheat cereal
Peanuts	Avocado	Wheat germ
Cashews	Broccoli	

POTASSIUM DEFICIENCY

Potassium is an important mineral. Your body needs potassium for many bodily functions, such as the regulation of fluid balance and blood pressure and the heart's electrical activity. Some types of cancer treatment, medications, and diarrhea can make your body lose potassium. If that's the case, your doctor or registered dietitian may recommend that you eat foods rich in potassium to help your blood levels get back to a healthy range.

GOOD SOURCES OF POTASSIUM

Avocado	Chocolate milk	Cooked Brussels sprouts
Banana	Milk	Spinach
Prunes	Yogurt (plain or with fruit)	Pork
Prune juice	Sweet potato	Halibut, tuna, cod, or salmon
Dates	Potatoes	
Figs	Cooked beets	

WEIGHT GAIN DURING TREATMENT

While most people undergoing cancer treatment lose weight, that's not the case for everyone. Some people gain weight during treatment. Hormone therapy, steroids, and some chemotherapy regimens can contribute to weight gain. Other treatments can cause fatigue or an increase in appetite, which could lead to weight gain.

If you notice you're gaining weight, talk with your health care team. They can help you determine the best way to proceed. These suggestions can help prevent unwanted weight gain:

- Talk to your doctor about being physically active during treatment, and try to avoid inactivity as best you can. There may be days when you don't feel like doing much, but try to incorporate some type of enjoyable physical activity most days of the week. For example, start walking five to ten minutes a day and work up to at least thirty minutes a day at a moderate pace. A moderate pace means that you are still able to talk while walking briskly. Other ideas include dancing, biking, yoga, and pilates.

- Limit how many sugary foods and drinks you consume. These foods contribute calories without nutrients.

- Choose lean sources of protein, such as fish, poultry, beans, and legumes.

- Limit your overall fat intake to help cut back on calories. Focus on healthy fats such as nuts and seeds and fatty fish (such as salmon, mackerel, tuna, and sardines).

- Increase the amount of fiber in your diet. High-fiber foods include vegetables and fruit with the peel left on, whole grains, nuts, and beans or peas. Check with your doctor first; fiber should be restricted for some people.

- Decrease your portion sizes, especially for high-fat foods and foods made with white (refined) flour and simple sugars.

- Do not skip meals, and try to eat your largest meal earlier in the day. It is okay to have snacks as long as they are healthy and you don't eat more overall.

- Pay attention to what triggers you to eat, and think about whether you are eating because of stress, boredom, or to meet an emotional need.

Aggressive weight loss is not typically recommended during treatment. It is best to discuss weight loss goals with your health care team and make a plan together.

NOTES

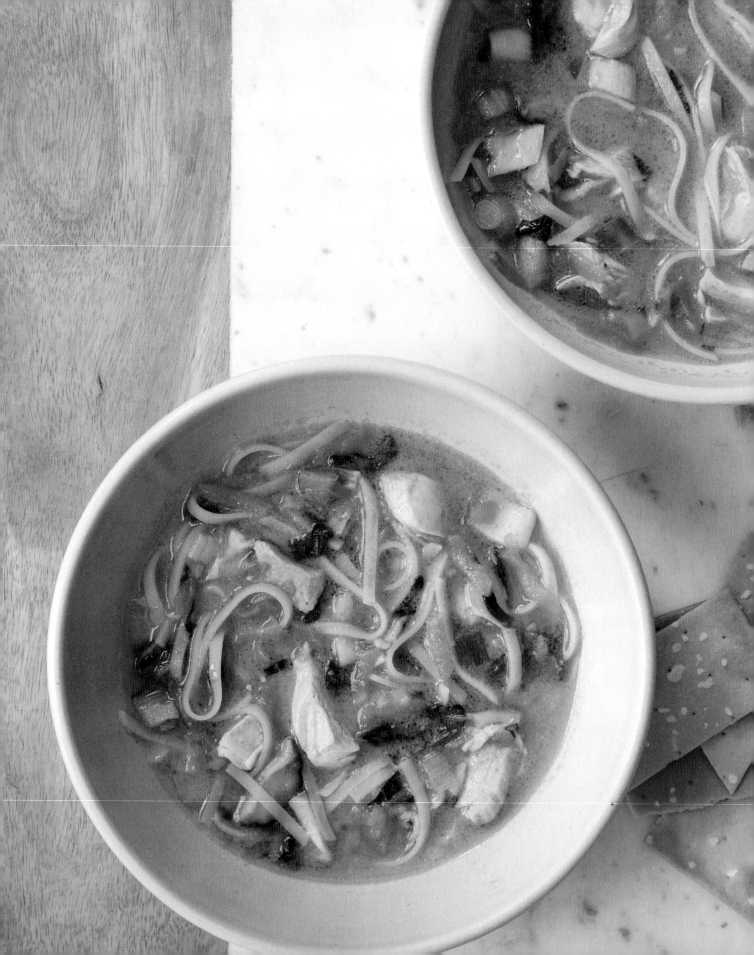

N NAUSEA

Carrot-Ginger Drink

Skillet Chicken with Root Vegetables

Quinoa–Sweet Potato Patties

Spring Minestrone

Chicken Broth Two Ways

Egg Roll-Up with Parsley and Dill

Mini Muffin Tin Chicken-Ricotta Meatballs

Pineapple-Mango Slushies

Steamed Chicken with Vegetables and Rice

Pumpkin-Ginger Mini Muffins

One-Bowl Gluten-Free Banana Pancakes

Miso-Chicken Soup

Ginger-Lime Spritzer

Blueberry-Corn Mini Muffins

Lemon-Ginger Biscotti

Mushroom Broth

On-the-Go Snack Mix

Strawberry-Watermelon-Mint Cooler

Chicken Noodle Soup

YOU MAY EXPERIENCE NAUSEA AND VOMITING WHILE YOU ARE GOING THROUGH CANCER TREATMENT. Nausea is the feeling of being queasy or sick to your stomach and can happen with or without vomiting. These side effects can vary widely and depend on the person and the type of treatment received. Some people going through cancer treatment have nausea and vomiting, while others have only nausea. Others have neither.

The most common causes of nausea and vomiting are chemotherapy and radiation therapy to the stomach, abdomen, or brain. Other causes of nausea and vomiting may include recovery from cancer-related surgery, pain, medications, illness, or being overly tired or anxious.

If your cancer treatment is causing nausea or vomiting, controlling it with the proper medication is very important. If you are prescribed anti-nausea medication, take it as directed. Many anti-nausea medications are meant to be taken on a schedule, not just when nausea occurs. If you are taking medicine as directed and are still nauseated, talk to your doctor about whether a different medication might be more beneficial. No matter the cause of your nausea and vomiting, this may be a time of trial and error as you and your doctor work to find the best way to deal with these side effects.

Managing Vomiting

If you are vomiting and cannot keep liquids down, dehydration can occur easily. Though it may be difficult, try to take in small amounts of liquid throughout the day to keep your body hydrated. Try sucking on ice chips or juice bars; eating small amounts of gelatin, sherbet, fruit ices, or slushies; or sipping clear liquids such as water, fruit juices (like apple or white grape juice), cool broths, sports drinks (oral rehydration drinks), coconut water, decaffeinated or herbal teas, and decaffeinated sodas (like ginger ale and lemon-lime) that have gone flat. Your doctor may be able to prescribe medicines in the form of dissolving tablets or suppositories.

Managing Nausea

Here are some tips that may help you manage nausea:

- Eat a small, light meal or snack before chemotherapy treatment.

- Focus on bland, easy-to-digest foods on scheduled treatment days.

- Sip on cool, cold, or room temperature clear liquids in small amounts.

- Keep something in your stomach by eating small, frequent snacks throughout the day—about every three hours. Snack ideas include smoothies, trail mix, fruit, or half a sandwich.

- Try starchy foods like pretzels, crackers, noodles, rice, potatoes, bagels, cereal, and toast.

- Eat food cool or cold to decrease its smell and taste. Sometimes strong odors and tastes can trigger nausea.

- Suck on frozen fruit, such as watermelon, peaches, grapes, berries, and cherries or tart hard candies, such as lemon drops (unless they irritate your mouth).

- Avoid eating your favorite foods when you do not feel well. If you eat your favorite foods when you are nauseated, you may associate them with feeling sick and find them unappealing when treatment is over.

- Avoid high-fat, greasy, spicy, and overly sweet foods.

- Tart or sour foods may be easier to keep down (but avoid if you have mouth sores).

- Try to rest quietly while sitting upright for at least an hour after each meal.

- Distract yourself with soft music, a favorite TV program, or the company of others.

- Avoid taking medications (especially pain medications) on an empty stomach unless the pharmacist directs you otherwise.

- Keep your mouth clean. Brush your teeth (with a soft bristle toothbrush) and rinse your mouth frequently with the homemade mouth rinse found on page 160 of this book.

- If your nausea is triggered by overtiredness or anxiety, ask your health care team for ideas for relaxation or coping techniques.

Managing Sensitivity to Smells

Smells can trigger nausea in some people or make it worse. People may not be aware that smells can make nausea worse. If certain smells bother you (such as perfumes, colognes, air fresheners, candles, etc.), explain their effect and ask for others' understanding. These additional tips can help you manage nausea caused by food or other aromas:

THE CLEAR LIQUID DIET

Clear liquids typically contain a small amount of calories and some electrolytes (sodium and potassium). Clear liquids are easy to digest and contain almost no fiber. These foods are typically allowed in a clear liquid diet:

Water (plain, carbonated, or flavored)

Clear fruit juices, such as white grape, cranberry, cranberry-apple, apple

Lemonade, limeade, and orange juice that is strained, with no pulp remaining

Clear sports drinks

Oral rehydration solutions (see recipes on pages 70–71)

Clear carbonated beverages, such as lemon-lime soda or ginger ale

Clear protein-containing nutrition supplements, such as Ensure Enlive or Boost Breeze

Broth, bouillon, or consommé

Decaffeinated or herbal tea

Decaffeinated coffee with no milk or cream (honey and sugar are okay)

Gelatin

Fruit ices made without fruit chunks or milk

Popsicles or frozen ice pops

Clear hard candy, such as lemon drops, root beer barrels, lollipops

- If the smell of food bothers you, try eating cold foods. Foods that are served cool or cold often have less odor and are milder tasting. In contrast, foods served hot or simmering often have stronger odors.

- Choose foods that do not need to be cooked, such as cereal and milk, cheese and crackers, a sandwich, gelatin, or pudding.

- Reheat foods in the microwave where cooking odors are contained, rather than simmering or cooking foods on top of the stove. Go to a different part of the house when cooking is happening, or ask others preparing food in your home to grill outdoors or use a slow cooker on the back porch or in the garage.

- Try using a straw for cold drinks or a covered cup or mug for soups to block odors.

- Eat in a well-ventilated area. Avoid eating in rooms that are stuffy or too warm. If someone else is cooking for you or bringing food, ask that they remove any food covers to release aromas before entering your room or eating area.

CONTACT YOUR DOCTOR IN THESE SITUATIONS:

- You vomit blood or material that looks like coffee grounds.

- You think you have inhaled vomit.

- You vomit more than three times an hour for three or more hours.

- You cannot consume more than four cups of liquid or ice chips in a 24-hour period.

- You are unable to eat food for more than two days.

- You are weak, lightheaded, or dizzy when changing position or standing up.

- You are unable to take medications as directed.

For more information about managing nausea and vomiting, visit the American Cancer Society website at cancer.org or call 800-227-2345.

Carrot–Ginger Drink

Carrots and ginger go well together, whether in a soup or a refreshing drink, such as this one. This dynamic duo is joined here with an orange for sweetness and cashews for surprising creaminess and added protein. This recipe will work best using a high-powered blender, such as a Vitamix, because puréeing raw vegetables and pulverizing nuts can overwhelm a standard blender's motor. If your blender isn't up to the task and you don't want to upgrade, try borrowing a friend's.

For food safety, use pasteurized cider rather than a raw or unpasteurized version you might buy from a farm stand.

2 SERVINGS

½ cup pasteurized apple cider or 100 percent apple juice

Juice of ½ lemon

1 orange, peeled and quartered

3 medium carrots, cut into 1-inch pieces

1 (½-inch) piece ginger, peeled and coarsely chopped

¼ cup roasted unsalted cashews

1 cup ice cubes

In a high-powered blender, combine the apple cider, lemon juice, orange, carrots, ginger, cashews, and ice cubes. Start on low and increase to high speed for 30 to 60 seconds, or until smooth.

PER SERVING

Calories	200
Fat	8 g
Saturated fat	1.5 g
Cholesterol	0 mg
Sodium	70 mg
Carbohydrate	31 g
Dietary fiber	5 g
Sugars	19 g
Protein	4 g
Calcium	80 mg
Potassium	610 mg

TIP For better blending, add liquids first and softer foods before more dense ingredients.

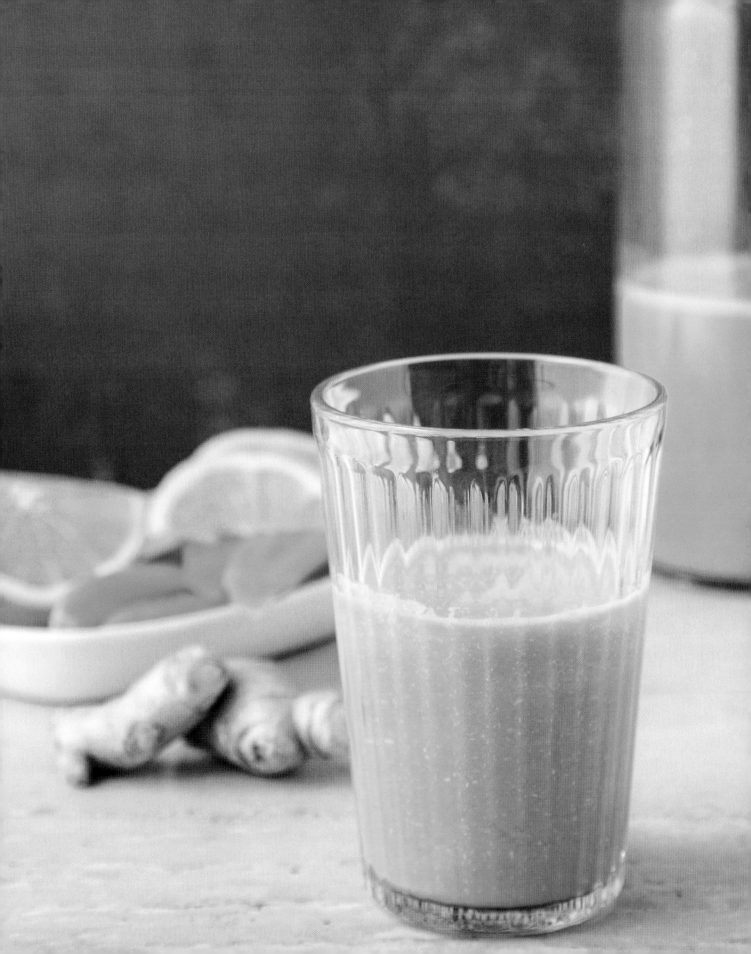

Skillet Chicken with Root Vegetables

This mild meal of braised chicken and meltingly soft root vegetables has comfort written all over it. As the mixture simmers, the chicken broth becomes infused with its flavors and transforms into a light but deeply satisfying sauce.

Try to cut the vegetables into uniformly sized pieces so they cook evenly. Because parsnips are often much thicker at the root end, you might need to quarter those sections. Peel the potatoes, parsnips, and carrots to make them easier to digest.

4 SERVINGS

4 boneless, skinless chicken breasts, pounded or sliced to even thickness

Salt and freshly ground black pepper

2 tablespoons olive oil, divided use

1 leek, white and light green parts only, thickly sliced

2 garlic cloves, minced

2 ½ cups homemade chicken broth (page 40) or store-bought reduced-sodium broth

8 new potatoes, halved

4 parsnips, cut into 1-inch pieces

4 carrots, cut into 1-inch pieces

2 fresh thyme sprigs, or 1 teaspoon dried thyme

Sprinkle the chicken with salt and pepper.

In a large skillet over medium-high heat, add 1 tablespoon of the oil. Cook the chicken for 3 to 5 minutes per side, or until cooked through and golden brown. Remove the chicken and set aside.

In the same skillet, add the remaining 1 tablespoon of oil and sauté the leeks for 3 to 5 minutes, or until softened. Add the garlic and sauté for 1 minute. Add the broth and bring to a boil, stirring to dislodge any bits of food that might have stuck to the bottom of the skillet. Reduce the heat, add the potatoes, parsnips, carrots, and thyme, and stir to distribute evenly. Cover and simmer for 15 minutes, or until the vegetables are tender. Return the chicken and any accumulated juices to the skillet, cover, and cook for 1 to 2 minutes, or until the chicken is heated through. Discard the thyme sprigs. Season with salt and pepper.

PER SERVING

Calories	400
Fat	11 g
Saturated fat	2 g
Cholesterol	70 mg
Sodium	430 mg
Carbohydrate	48 g
Dietary fiber	8 g
Sugars	9 g
Protein	29 g
Calcium	100 mg
Potassium	1220 mg

TIP For better browning, pat chicken dry with paper towels before searing. Rinsing raw chicken is actually not recommended—splashing water increases the risk of spreading bacteria. Proper cooking will kill the bacteria.

Quinoa–Sweet Potato Patties

These mildly flavored, baked vegetarian "burgers" can be eaten on a bun or on their own. For smaller appetites, make twelve patties instead of six larger ones and keep them on hand for snacking during the day (if making smaller patties, shorten the baking time by five to ten minutes).

These patties pack a big nutritional punch! Quinoa is a great source of protein and magnesium, and sweet potatoes are loaded with beta carotene.

6 SERVINGS

1 cup quinoa

1 tablespoon finely chopped shallot

1 cup finely chopped fresh spinach leaves

1 egg

1 cup mashed sweet potato

1 tablespoon white or red wine vinegar

½ cup plain bread crumbs

1 teaspoon salt

Preheat the oven to 400 degrees.

Prepare the quinoa according to the package directions, adding the shallot after the water comes to a boil. When the quinoa has finished cooking, add the spinach and stir until softened and combined.

Meanwhile, in a large bowl, beat the egg. Add the sweet potato and vinegar and stir to combine. Add the bread crumbs and salt and stir to combine. Add the quinoa mixture and stir to combine.

Form the mixture into six ¾-inch-thick patties (lightly wet your hands if the mixture is sticking to them). Place the patties on a baking sheet and bake for 25 minutes, flipping the burgers after 15 minutes.

PER SERVING (ONE PATTY)	
Calories	190
Fat	3 g
Saturated fat	0.5 g
Cholesterol	30 mg
Sodium	490 mg
Carbohydrate	34 g
Dietary fiber	4 g
Sugars	5 g
Protein	7 g
Calcium	60 mg
Potassium	410 mg

TIP If you don't have leftover cooked sweet potato, microwave a small one (seven to eight minutes should do it) while the quinoa cooks.

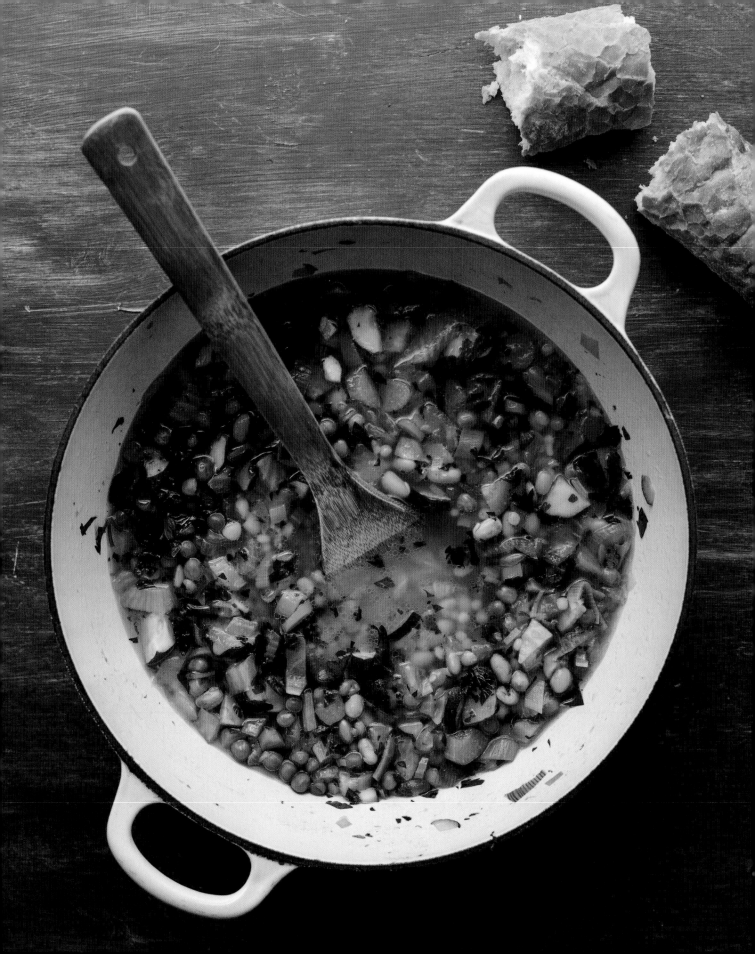

Spring Minestrone

In warmer months, a light vegetable soup highlighting fresh flavors from the garden is highly desirable. This soup doesn't skimp on the veggies or legumes. Edamame (green soybeans often served at Japanese restaurants) provide added protein, fiber, and many other nutrients. A flurry of fresh herbs provides aromatic endnotes, and a splash of lemon juice adds a bright hint of spring.

This is a "vegetable-centric" soup. If you want a thinner version, add one to two more cups of broth.

4 SERVINGS

¼ cup ditalini, pastina, or other tiny pasta

2 tablespoons olive oil

1 leek, white and light green parts only, quartered lengthwise and sliced

1 small onion, finely chopped

1 carrot, chopped

1 celery stalk, chopped

1 small zucchini, chopped

½ fennel bulb, cored and chopped

1 garlic clove, minced

4 cups homemade chicken or vegetable broth (pages 40 or 74) or store-bought reduced-sodium broth

1 cup canned navy beans, rinsed and drained

½ cup frozen peas

½ cup frozen shelled edamame

Salt and freshly ground black pepper

½ cup chopped fresh Italian parsley

¼ cup chopped fresh basil leaves

1 tablespoon fresh lemon juice, optional

Prepare the pasta according to the package directions for al dente (just firm). Drain and set aside.

Meanwhile, in a large stockpot over medium heat, add the oil. Sauté the leek, onion, carrot, celery, zucchini, and fennel for 8 to 10 minutes, or until softened. Add the garlic and sauté for 1 minute. Add the broth and bring to a boil, stirring to combine. Reduce the heat, cover, and simmer for 10 to 15 minutes, or until the vegetables are tender. Add the navy beans, peas, edamame, and reserved pasta, and stir to combine. Season with salt and pepper. Add the parsley, basil, and lemon juice, if desired.

PER SERVING	
Calories	260
Fat	9 g
Saturated fat	1.5 g
Cholesterol	5 mg
Sodium	650 mg
Carbohydrate	35 g
Dietary fiber	10 g
Sugars	6 g
Protein	12 g
Calcium	120 mg
Potassium	710 mg

TIP For the family (or when the side effect has resolved), swirl a dab of prepared pesto into the soup or top with freshly grated Parmesan cheese for more assertive flavor.

Chicken Broth Two Ways

Homemade broth is preservative free, economical, and allows you to control how much sodium you use. It isn't as much of a chore as you might think when using a slow cooker (Crock Pot). Just combine the ingredients in the morning and let it simmer on low the whole day. If time allows, make it a day ahead and refrigerate overnight so that you can easily skim the fat from the top.

Many stores sell meaty backs and other bones for a fraction of the cost of a whole chicken. If you don't see them, ask the butcher to put some aside for you. Chicken wings can also be used.

For a richer flavor to sip on or use in a chicken-based soup, such as chicken noodle, roast the bones first. Use the lighter version for general cooking.

Refrigerate until ready to use or eat. Freeze unused broth in quart containers for later use.

Light Chicken Broth

Just combine and step away! It doesn't get any easier than that.

MAKES 3 QUARTS

3 pounds meaty chicken bones and/or wings

1 onion, quartered

1 garlic clove, smashed

1 to 2 tablespoons salt

5 black peppercorns

3 quarts water

Freshly ground black pepper

In a slow cooker, combine the bones, onion, garlic, 1 tablespoon of the salt, and peppercorns. Add the water to cover. Cook on low for 8 to 10 hours or high for 4 to 5, or until you can smell a rich cooked poultry aroma. Set aside to cool.

Place a large strainer in a large bowl and carefully transfer the contents of the pot to the strainer, pushing down with a spoon to extract all the liquid. Discard the solids. Season with additional salt and pepper. If time allows, refrigerate to let the fat rise to the top and skim before using.

PER SERVING

Calories	15
Fat	1 g
Saturated fat	0 g
Cholesterol	5 mg
Sodium	500 mg
Carbohydrate	0 g
Dietary fiber	0 g
Sugars	0 g
Protein	2 g
Calcium	9 mg
Potassium	15 mg

Dark Roasted Chicken Broth

Roasting the chicken bones before adding them to the slow cooker coaxes out deeper flavor. The heat from the oven causes the bones to caramelize, which will make a richer broth. Another plus—most of the fat will melt into the pan during baking, eliminating the need to skim it after making the broth. Line the pan with foil for easier cleanup.

MAKES 3 QUARTS

3 pounds meaty chicken bones and/or wings

2 teaspoons canola oil

1 onion, quartered

1 garlic clove, smashed

1 to 2 tablespoons salt

5 black peppercorns

3 quarts water

Freshly ground black pepper

Preheat the oven to 375 degrees.

In a roasting pan, place the bones and drizzle with oil. Bake for 1 to 1 ½ hours, or until the bones are golden brown.

Transfer the bones to a slow cooker, discarding the excess fat in the pan. Add the onion, garlic, 1 tablespoon of the salt, and peppercorns. Add the water to cover. Cook on low for 8 to 10 hours or high for 4 to 5, or until you can smell a rich poultry aroma. Set aside to cool.

Place a large strainer in a large bowl and carefully transfer the contents of the pot to the strainer, pushing down with a spoon to extract all the liquid. Season with additional salt and pepper. Discard the solids.

PER SERVING

Calories	25
Fat	1.5 g
Saturated fat	0 g
Cholesterol	5 mg
Sodium	500 mg
Carbohydrate	0 g
Dietary fiber	0 g
Sugars	0 g
Protein	2 g
Calcium	9 mg
Potassium	15 mg

Egg Roll-Up with Parsley and Dill

When appetites are small, a crêpe-like omelet flecked with fresh herbs provides healthy nourishment in a jiffy. Cook, roll, and you are ready to go!

If your stomach can handle something a little heavier, spoon a tablespoon or so of cottage cheese on the cooked egg before rolling for added protein, or wrap the egg in a small tortilla after rolling.

If flipping the omelet over in the pan seems daunting, slide it out onto a plate, cooked side down, and invert the plate over the pan to finish cooking the second side of the egg.

1 SERVING

1 egg

1 teaspoon finely chopped fresh Italian parsley

1/2 teaspoon finely chopped fresh dill

Salt and freshly ground black pepper

In a bowl, beat the egg, parsley, and dill and sprinkle with salt and pepper.

Lightly coat an 8- or 10-inch, preferably nonstick, skillet with nonstick cooking spray and place over medium heat. Add the egg and swirl it around like a crêpe so that it forms a thin layer in the pan. Cook without stirring for 20 to 30 seconds, or until it is set on the bottom. Using a spatula, flip the egg and cook for 20 to 30 seconds, or until set on both sides. Using a spatula, or your fingers, roll the egg up into a cylinder for easy eating.

PER SERVING	
Calories	70
Fat	5 g
Saturated fat	1.5 g
Cholesterol	185 mg
Sodium	70 mg
Carbohydrate	0 g
Dietary fiber	0 g
Sugars	0 g
Protein	6 g
Calcium	30 mg
Potassium	75 mg

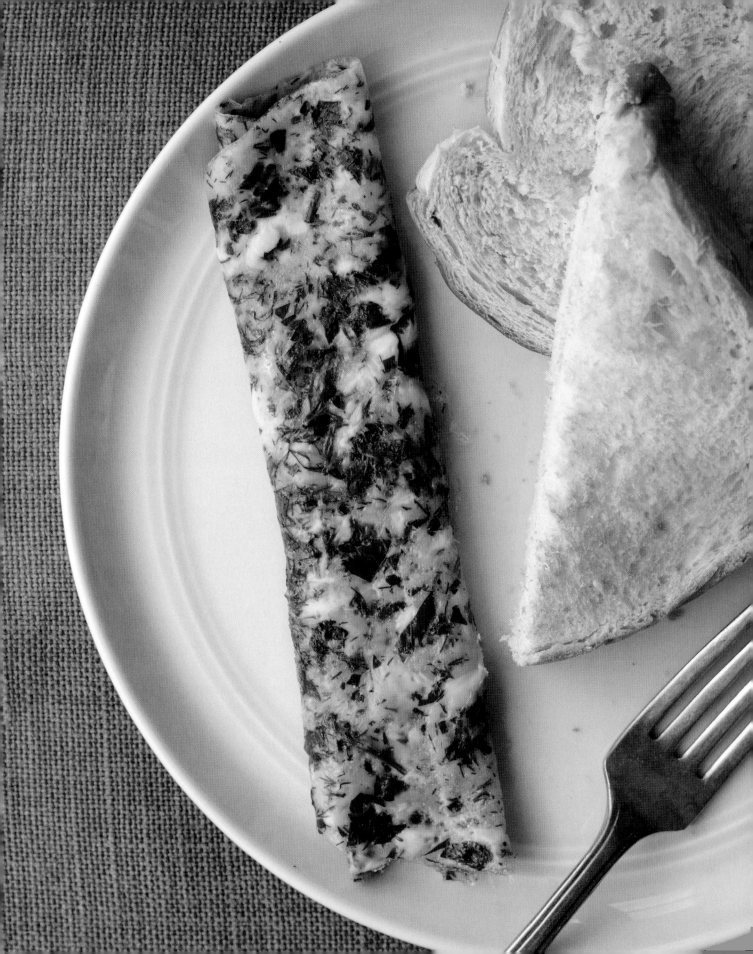

Mini Muffin Tin Chicken-Ricotta Meatballs

These mild chicken meatballs are great to have on hand for dinner or a snack when hunger strikes. If you're going out and will be missing a meal, put a few in a cooler and take them with you for nibbling.

Using a mini muffin tin makes prep a snap: with no need to roll the mixture into balls, you simply fill the cups and gently pat the tops. If you can handle more flavor, add a minced garlic clove. If you don't have a mini muffin tin, roll into twenty-four meatballs and bake until cooked through.

Because fat can aggravate nausea, use reduced-fat ricotta cheese here.

MAKES 24 MEATBALLS

1 egg

1 pound ground chicken

1/2 cup reduced-fat ricotta cheese

1/4 cup panko or dried bread crumbs

1/4 cup freshly grated Parmesan cheese

2 tablespoons finely chopped onion

2 tablespoons chopped fresh Italian parsley

Salt and freshly ground black pepper

Preheat the oven to 400 degrees. Coat one (24-hole) or two (12-hole) mini muffin tins with nonstick cooking spray.

In a bowl, beat the egg. Add the chicken and gently stir to combine. Add the ricotta cheese, panko, Parmesan, onion, and parsley. Sprinkle with salt and pepper and gently stir to combine. Drop tablespoons of the mixture into the muffin cups. Using a wet finger, smooth the tops of the meatballs. Bake for 14 to 16 minutes, or until firm and cooked through.

PER SERVING (ONE MEATBALL)	
Calories	35
Fat	1 g
Saturated fat	0.5 g
Cholesterol	25 mg
Sodium	40 mg
Carbohydrate	1 g
Dietary fiber	0 g
Sugars	0 g
Protein	5 g
Calcium	20 mg
Potassium	60 mg

TIP For the family (or when the side effect has resolved), dip meatballs into your favorite marinara sauce or make a dipping sauce with 1/4 cup reduced-fat mayonnaise, 2 tablespoons apricot jam, and 1 tablespoon Dijon mustard.

Pineapple–Mango Slushies

To make this easy, frosty treat, simply freeze the juice and fruit mixture and, right before serving, purée in the food processor until it has a soft and slushy texture. You can use any flavor of juice that sounds appealing or try other fruits in place of the pineapple.

You can also use this recipe to make fruit pops. Cover each paper cup with a piece of plastic wrap or aluminum foil and make a slit in the wrap. Insert a plastic spoon or Popsicle stick through the wrap and freeze until the fruit mixture is solid, at least three hours.

Avoid this recipe if you have a sore mouth or throat.

4 SERVINGS

1 (8-ounce) can crushed pineapple in juice

3 cups mango-pineapple or other tropical fruit juice, divided use

In four (¾- to 1-cup) paper cups, divide pineapple evenly (about ¼ cup per cup). Fill each cup with ½ cup of the juice and stir to combine. Cover each cup with plastic wrap and freeze until solid, at least 3 hours.

Remove the frozen mixture from the cups by running the outside of the cup under hot water and peeling off the paper. Place the frozen pops (one at a time) in a food processor with ¼ cup juice and process until slushy.

PER SERVING	
Calories	130
Fat	0 g
Saturated fat	0 g
Cholesterol	0 mg
Sodium	25 mg
Carbohydrate	30 g
Dietary fiber	0.5 g
Sugars	30 g
Protein	0 g
Calcium	40 mg
Potassium	110 mg

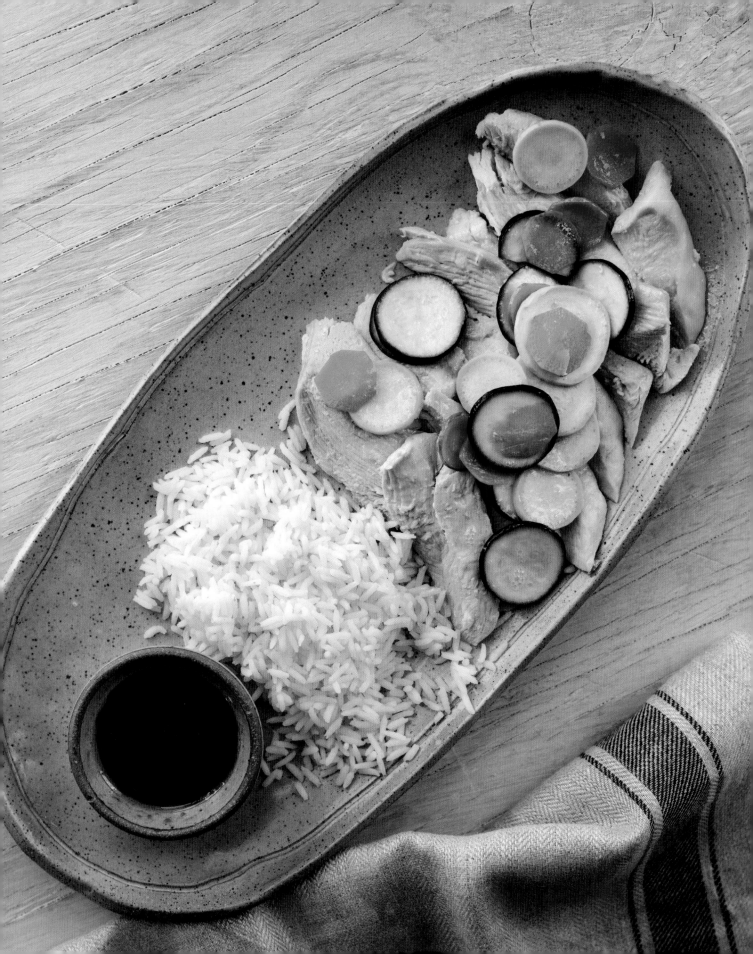

Steamed Chicken with Vegetables and Rice

When your stomach is feeling delicate, this dish of simple steamed chicken and mildly flavored vegetables provides gentle sustenance and beneficial nutrients. Adding lemon slices to the steaming liquid subtly infuses the chicken with flavor while it cooks. For added flavor, substitute chicken broth for the water when preparing the rice.

If you are up to it, add a dipping sauce to drizzle over the chicken. Combine two tablespoons reduced-sodium soy sauce or tamari, one tablespoon rice vinegar, one tablespoon mirin, two teaspoons honey, and one teaspoon dark sesame oil.

For a more modern spin, wrap the chicken and veggies in a tortilla or lettuce leaf (if you're not having diarrhea) and eat like a taco.

4 SERVINGS

1 cup basmati or other rice, rinsed

1 lemon, thinly sliced

1 pound boneless, skinless chicken breasts, cut into 1-inch "strips"

Salt and freshly ground black pepper

1 carrot, thinly sliced

1 zucchini, thinly sliced

1 yellow squash, thinly sliced

Prepare the rice according to the package directions.

Meanwhile, in a stockpot, place the lemon slices in 1 to 2 inches of water (the water shouldn't reach the steamer). Bring the water to a boil, then reduce the heat to a simmer.

Lightly coat a steamer basket with nonstick cooking spray. Sprinkle the chicken with salt and pepper, place it in a single layer in the steamer basket, and top with the carrot. Set the basket in the stockpot over the simmering water. Cover and cook for 8 minutes. Add the zucchini and squash slices. Cover and cook for 5 minutes, or until the chicken is cooked through and the vegetables are tender. Serve the chicken and vegetables with the rice.

PER SERVING

Calories	300
Fat	3.5 g
Saturated fat	1 g
Cholesterol	65 mg
Sodium	75 mg
Carbohydrate	39 g
Dietary fiber	2 g
Sugars	3 g
Protein	28 g
Calcium	40 mg
Potassium	540 mg

TIP A pasta pot with an insert for steaming works well for making this dish. A mandoline or food processor with a slicing blade cuts the vegetables thinly in a jiffy.

Pumpkin-Ginger Mini Muffins

These delicately spiced muffins get extra flavor and texture from currants (perfectly sized for miniature treats) and crystallized ginger, available in the baking section of most supermarkets. To make these muffins extra mild, you can leave out the crystallized ginger.

To make regular-sized muffins, add five to ten minutes to the baking time. This recipe makes about a dozen regular-sized muffins.

24 MINI MUFFINS

1 cup all-purpose flour

1/2 cup granulated sugar

1 teaspoon baking powder

1/4 teaspoon baking soda

1/4 teaspoon salt

1/2 teaspoon ground cinnamon

1/2 teaspoon ground ginger

Pinch ground nutmeg

Pinch ground cloves

1/4 cup currants, golden raisins, or brown raisins

2 tablespoons finely chopped crystallized ginger

1 egg

1/4 cup butter, melted and slightly cooled

3 tablespoons water

1/2 cup canned pumpkin purée

Preheat the oven to 350 degrees. Coat two mini muffin tins with nonstick cooking spray or fill with paper liners.

In a bowl, combine flour, sugar, baking powder, baking soda, salt, cinnamon, ground ginger, nutmeg, and cloves. Add the currants and crystallized ginger and stir gently to coat.

In a separate bowl, beat the egg. Add the butter, water, and pumpkin and stir to combine. Add the egg mixture to the dry ingredients and stir gently to incorporate. Spoon the batter evenly into muffin cups.

Bake for 12 to 15 minutes, or until the tops just bounce back when touched. Leave in the tins for 5 to 10 minutes before transferring to a cooling rack.

PER SERVING
(ONE MINI MUFFIN)

Calories	70
Fat	2 g
Saturated fat	1.5 g
Cholesterol	15 mg
Sodium	70 mg
Carbohydrate	11 g
Dietary fiber	0 g
Sugars	6 g
Protein	1 g
Calcium	20 mg
Potassium	40 mg

 TIP For stronger flavor, increase the amounts of the ground spices.

One-Bowl Gluten-Free Banana Pancakes

Tasty and fast, these gluten-free, four-ingredient pancakes are appropriate for breakfast or a snack.

To test whether the skillet is hot enough to prevent sticking, flick a bit of water into it—it should sizzle. Keep the pancakes the size of a silver dollar and use a thin, firm spatula, which will allow you to get under the pancakes easily to flip them.

2 SERVINGS

1 medium ripe banana

2 eggs, beaten well

⅛ teaspoon baking powder

Pinch salt

In a bowl, mash the banana until almost smooth. You should have ¼ to ⅓ cup. Add the eggs, baking powder, and salt and stir until combined. The batter will be very thin.

Preheat a griddle or skillet over medium heat and coat with nonstick cooking spray. Spoon 2 tablespoons of batter, 3 to 4 inches apart. You should be able to fit several at a time. Cook for 30 to 60 seconds or until golden on the bottom. Carefully flip the pancakes. If some batter spills during flipping, place the flipped pancake on top of the spilled batter. Repeat with the remaining batter.

PER SERVING

Calories	130
Fat	5 g
Saturated fat	1.5 g
Cholesterol	185 mg
Sodium	170 mg
Carbohydrate	15 g
Dietary fiber	2 g
Sugars	8 g
Protein	7 g
Calcium	50 mg
Potassium	300 mg

 TIP Serve with maple syrup, fruit compote, or peanut or almond butter for added calories.

Miso-Chicken Soup

Miso, a good-for-your-gut probiotic, is a product of fermented soybeans. It adds a unique savory flavor, known as umami. Umami is called the fifth taste, in addition to sweet, sour, bitter, and salty. It provides depth to this comforting, main-course, Asian-inspired chicken soup, which is flecked with mushrooms, carrots, and bok choy.

If you can't find low-sodium or unsalted broth, use five cups reduced-sodium broth and one cup water. If you'd like the soup to have a stronger miso flavor and be saltier, increase the amount of miso paste to taste.

4 TO 6 SERVINGS

4 ounces rice noodles

1 tablespoon canola oil

6 ounces shiitake mushrooms, stemmed and thinly sliced

4 scallions, white and light green parts only, thinly sliced

2 carrots, grated

2 garlic cloves, minced

1 tablespoon finely chopped fresh ginger

6 cups homemade chicken broth (page 40) or store-bought low-sodium or unsalted broth

3 tablespoons white miso paste

1 pound boneless, skinless chicken breasts, halved lengthwise and thinly sliced

2 heads baby bok choy (8 to 10 ounces), cored and thinly sliced

Prepare the noodles according to the package directions, drain, and set aside.

In a large stockpot over medium heat, add the oil. Sauté the mushrooms, scallions, carrots, garlic, and ginger for 5 to 8 minutes, or until softened. Add the broth and miso and bring to a boil. Reduce the heat and simmer for 10 minutes. Add the chicken and cook for 5 to 8 minutes, or until the chicken is cooked through, stirring occasionally. Add the reserved noodles and bok choy and cook for 1 to 2 minutes, or until the bok choy is bright green and the noodles are heated through.

PER SERVING

Calories	370
Fat	7 g
Saturated fat	1 g
Cholesterol	65 mg
Sodium	610 mg
Carbohydrate	37 g
Dietary fiber	4 g
Sugars	7 g
Protein	38 g
Calcium	120 mg
Potassium	890 mg

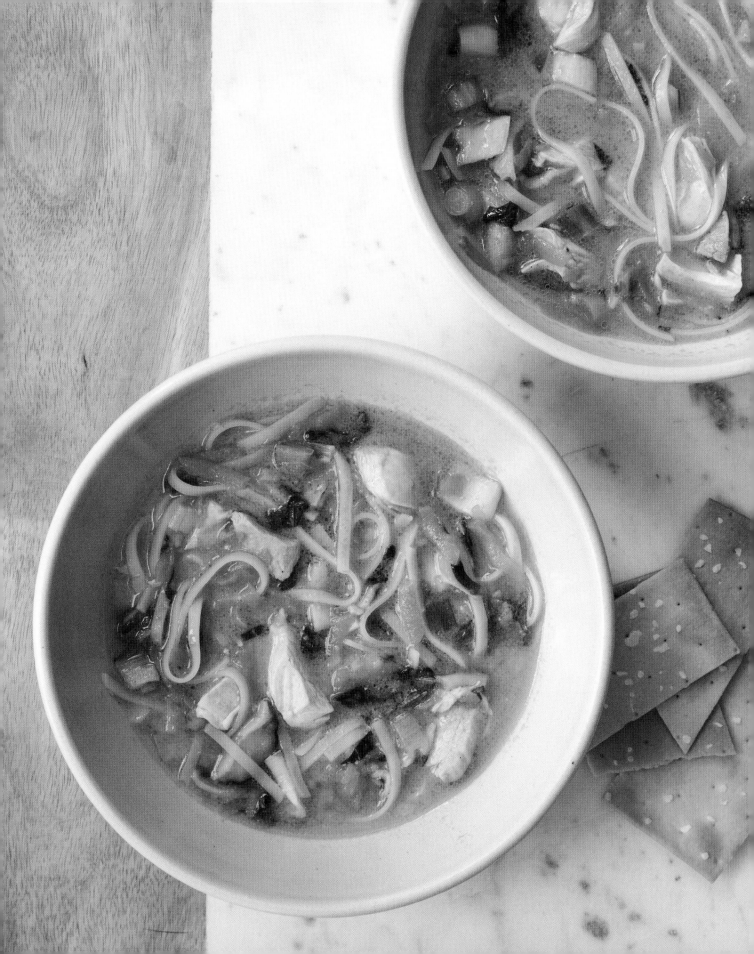

Ginger-Lime Spritzer

A simple syrup of equal parts water and sugar and lots of fresh ginger is the base of this refreshing drink, just right to sip on when you are feeling under the weather. A splash of "fizzy water" adds sparkle and can aid digestion for many.

5 SERVINGS

1 cup water

1 cup granulated sugar

¼ cup (2 ounces) peeled and chopped fresh ginger

5 cups seltzer, club soda, or sparkling water

Ice, optional

1 lime, cut into 5 wedges, optional

In a saucepan over medium-high heat, combine the water and sugar and bring to a boil, swirling the mixture until the sugar completely dissolves. Stir in the ginger and remove from the heat. Set aside for 1 hour. Strain the ginger syrup into a container or bowl, pushing down with a spoon to extract all the liquid, and refrigerate until ready to use.

In a glass, add ¼ cup ginger syrup and 1 cup seltzer, or to taste. Add ice and a wedge of lime, if desired.

PER SERVING	
Calories	160
Fat	0 g
Saturated fat	0 g
Cholesterol	0 mg
Sodium	55 mg
Carbohydrate	42 g
Dietary fiber	0 g
Sugars	40 g
Protein	0 g
Calcium	20 mg
Potassium	50 mg

 TIP You can also use the ginger syrup to add flavor to other foods. Drizzle it over fruit salad, citrus slices, or plain yogurt.

Blueberry-Corn Mini Muffins

These not-too-sweet muffins provide antioxidants through the addition of blueberries. If using frozen berries, use small ones and do not defrost first.

Coating the blueberries with a little flour keeps them more evenly distributed in the batter.

To make regular-sized muffins, add five to ten minutes to the baking time. This recipe should make about twelve regular-sized muffins.

24 MINI MUFFINS

3/4 cup cornmeal

1/4 cup all-purpose flour

3 tablespoons granulated sugar

1 1/4 teaspoons baking powder

1/2 teaspoon salt

1 cup fresh or frozen blueberries

1 egg

3/4 cup buttermilk

1/4 cup canola oil

Preheat the oven to 400 degrees. Coat two mini muffin tins with nonstick cooking spray or fill with paper liners.

In a bowl, combine the cornmeal, flour, sugar, baking powder, and salt. Add the blueberries and stir gently to coat.

In a separate bowl, beat the egg. Add the buttermilk and oil and stir to combine. Add the egg mixture to the dry ingredients and stir gently to incorporate. Spoon the batter evenly into muffin cups.

Bake for 15 to 17 minutes, or until the tops just bounce back when touched. Leave in the tins for 5 to 10 minutes before transferring to a cooling rack.

PER SERVING
(ONE MINI MUFFIN)

Calories	60
Fat	2.5 g
Saturated fat	0 g
Cholesterol	10 mg
Sodium	80 mg
Carbohydrate	7 g
Dietary fiber	0 g
Sugars	3 g
Protein	1 g
Calcium	30 mg
Potassium	30 mg

 TIP If you don't have canola oil on hand, you can substitute another vegetable oil.

Lemon-Ginger Biscotti

If you feel like something a little sweet, try one of these biscotti. These have enough flavor to be appealing but not overpowering. The addition of both ground ginger and crystallized ginger makes for a double dose of its stomach-soothing properties.

28 BISCOTTI

2 cups all-purpose flour

1/2 cup finely chopped crystallized ginger

1 teaspoon baking powder

1 teaspoon ground ginger

1/2 teaspoon baking soda

1/4 teaspoon salt

2 eggs

2/3 cup granulated sugar

Zest of 1 lemon

1 tablespoon fresh lemon juice

Preheat the oven to 350 degrees. Line two baking sheets with parchment paper or foil.

In a bowl, combine the flour, crystallized ginger, baking powder, ground ginger, baking soda, and salt. Set aside.

In a bowl, using an electric mixer, beat the eggs, sugar, and lemon zest and juice for 1 minute, or until smooth and golden.

On low speed, gradually add the dry ingredients, scraping down the beater(s) and sides to blend. The dough will be dry and crumbly at first but then will begin to take form. Scrape the dough onto a work surface that has been lightly coated with flour. Lightly coat your hands with flour and knead briefly until dough is soft and not sticky (about eight to ten times).

Divide the dough into two pieces. Shape each piece into a cylinder about 10 inches long, 2 inches wide, and 1 inch high. Carefully transfer the logs to a baking sheet, placing them 4 inches apart. Bake for 35 to 40 minutes, or until well risen, golden, and firm to the touch. Remove from the oven and reduce the temperature to 325 degrees.

Cool the dough on the baking sheet for about 10 minutes, or until warm but not too hot to touch. Peel off the paper or foil and transfer the logs to a cutting board. Using a serrated or sharp knife, cut diagonal 1/2-inch-thick slices. Use a firm and fast cutting motion to prevent crumbling.

Lay the cut biscotti flat on the baking sheets. You will need two sheets to fit all of the biscotti. Return the baking sheets to the oven and bake until golden brown, firm, and dry, 20 to 25 minutes. The cookies might be slightly soft in the center but will harden as they cool. Let stand 2 minutes. Remove them from the baking sheet to a cooling rack.

PER SERVING (ONE BISCOTTI)	
Calories	70
Fat	0 g
Saturated fat	0 g
Cholesterol	15 mg
Sodium	60 mg
Carbohydrate	15 g
Dietary fiber	0 g
Sugars	7 g
Protein	1 g
Calcium	20 mg
Potassium	20 mg

TIP For extra-wide biscotti, shape the dough into a single 14-inch-long roll and flatten to 1 inch.

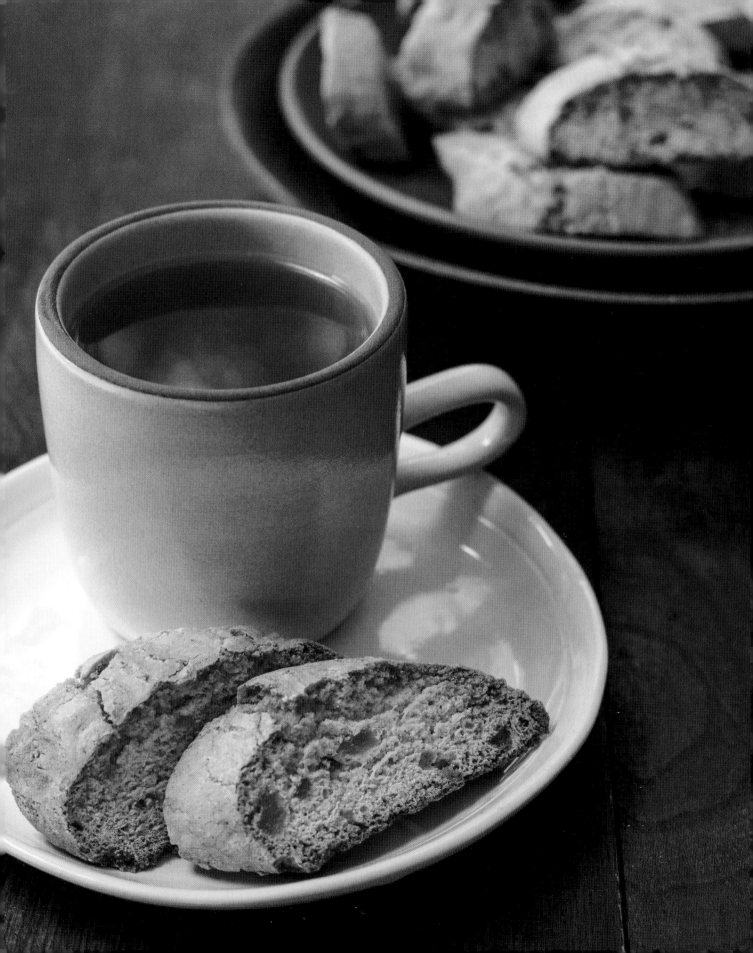

Mushroom Broth

When your stomach is sensitive and you want something warm and comforting, try this earthy broth.

You can add any of your favorite aromatics and use whatever mushrooms you have or can find at the market. Dried mushrooms will boost the flavor, but if you have trouble finding them, the broth will still be good with only fresh.

Use a food processor to quickly chop the vegetables; they don't need to be cut absolutely evenly when making broths.

4 SERVINGS

2 tablespoons olive oil

1 onion, coarsely chopped

1 celery stalk, coarsely chopped

1 carrot, coarsely chopped

1 leek, white and light green parts only, sliced

4 medium garlic cloves

1 pound white mushrooms, coarsely chopped

1/2 cup dried mushrooms, such as porcini or shiitake or a mixture

4 fresh Italian parsley sprigs

3 fresh thyme sprigs

1 bay leaf

1 teaspoon black peppercorns

8 cups water

2 tablespoons reduced-sodium soy sauce or tamari

In a large stockpot over medium heat, add the oil. Sauté the onion, celery, carrot, and leek for 8 to 10 minutes, or until softened. Add the garlic and mushrooms and sauté for 5 minutes, or until the mushrooms soften and release their liquid. Add the parsley, thyme, bay leaf, and peppercorns and stir to combine. Add the water and soy sauce and bring to a boil. Reduce the heat and simmer for 1 hour, or until the stock is reduced by about half. Set aside to cool briefly.

Place a large strainer in a large bowl or pot and carefully transfer the contents of the pot to the strainer, pushing down with a spoon to extract all the liquid. Discard the solids.

PER SERVING	
Calories	70
Fat	7 g
Saturated fat	1 g
Cholesterol	0 mg
Sodium	300 mg
Carbohydrate	2 g
Dietary fiber	0 g
Sugars	0.5 g
Protein	1 g
Calcium	20 mg
Potassium	70 mg

TIP Refrigerate until ready to use or eat. Freeze unused broth in quart containers to have on hand to use later.

On-the-Go Snack Mix

Snack mixes are handy to have preassembled for a quick snack. Keep the mix in a tightly sealed container in your bag or backpack, in the car, or by the couch.

You can adapt the ingredients depending on your symptoms. If you're experiencing constipation, include dried fruits and cereals with at least five grams of fiber, such as Mini Wheats or Wheat Chex. A sprinkling of nuts adds protein. And, of course, a little chocolate rarely hurts! If you are very nauseated, use a plainer cracker, such as Wheat Thins, and omit the M&M'S.

9 SERVINGS

1 cup pretzels

1 cup plain or peanut butter Ritz bits, Wheat Thins, or other small crackers

1 cup whole grain cereal, such as Cheerios or Quaker Oatmeal Squares

1/2 cup dry-roasted almonds

1/2 cup raisins

1/2 cup plain or peanut M&M'S, optional

In a container with an airtight lid, combine the pretzels, crackers, cereal, almonds, raisins, and M&M'S, if desired.

PER SERVING	
Calories	150
Fat	7 g
Saturated fat	1 g
Cholesterol	0 mg
Sodium	170 mg
Carbohydrate	19 g
Dietary fiber	2 g
Sugars	7 g
Protein	4 g
Calcium	40 mg
Potassium	170 mg

TIP Nuts provide protein and are relatively low in saturated fat.

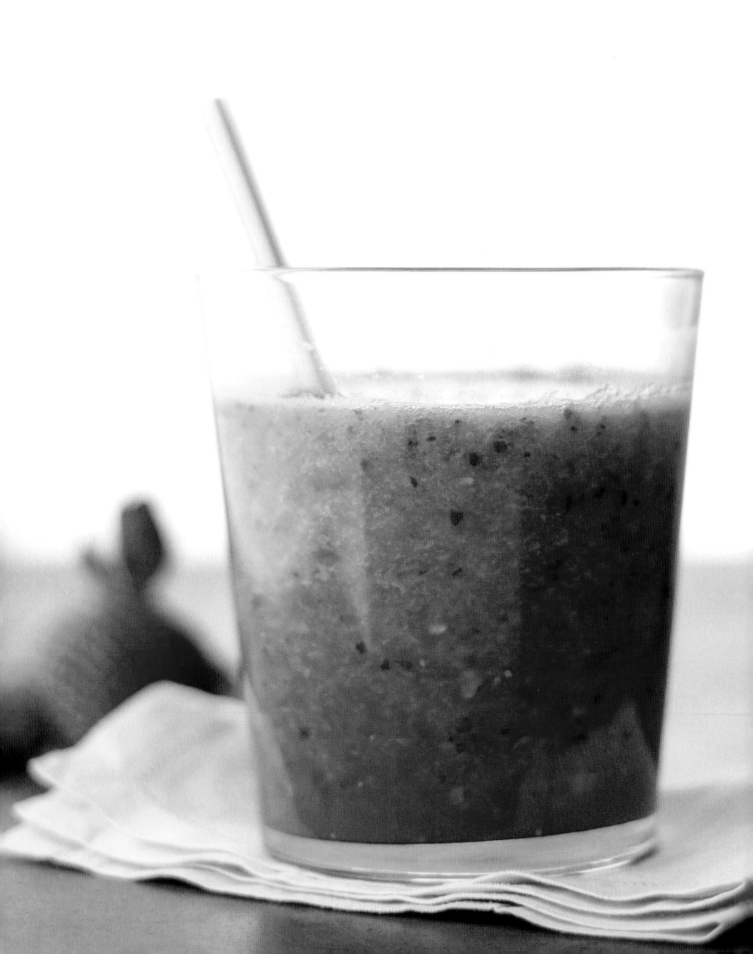

Strawberry-Watermelon-Mint Cooler

This cooling drink combines the flavors of everyone's favorite summer fruit with touches of herbal and citrus essence.

The frozen strawberries provide the drink's frosty texture. Make sure your watermelon is ripe and sweet for optimum flavor.

2 SERVINGS

2 cups seedless watermelon chunks, chilled

2 tablespoons chopped fresh mint leaves

1 to 2 tablespoons honey

1 teaspoon finely grated lemon zest, optional

1 cup frozen strawberries

In a blender, add the watermelon, mint, 1 tablespoon of the honey, and lemon zest, if desired, and blend until liquefied. Add the strawberries and blend until smooth. Taste and add honey, if desired.

PER SERVING

Calories	110
Fat	0 g
Saturated fat	0 g
Cholesterol	0 mg
Sodium	5 mg
Carbohydrate	27 g
Dietary fiber	3 g
Sugars	22 g
Protein	1 g
Calcium	30 mg
Potassium	310 mg

Chicken Noodle Soup

A store-bought rotisserie chicken is a mealtime lifesaver. It can be made into salads, sandwiches, or, as in this recipe, a classically loved soup.

This version uses all of the white breast meat from the chicken. Sautéing the wings and other bones with the aromatic vegetables adds richer flavor. If you prefer a less chunky soup, start with just one cup of chicken and add more to taste. If you want a thicker, noodle-filled broth, increase the amount of noodles in the recipe by one-half cup. Unused dark meat can be saved for another meal.

Avoid getting a rotisserie chicken that has been sitting out for very long. Try asking the deli staff if they can give you a fresh one or tell you which are the freshest in the warmer.

8 SERVINGS

1 rotisserie chicken full breast or 3 cups chopped cooked chicken

1 tablespoon canola oil

1 onion, chopped

1 large carrot (or 2 small), sliced

1 large celery stalk (or 2 small), sliced

6 cups homemade chicken broth (page 40) or store-bought reduced-sodium broth

2 cups water

½ cup egg noodles

2 tablespoons chopped fresh Italian parsley

Salt and freshly ground black pepper

Remove the wings from the chicken breast and reserve. Remove the skin from the breast and discard. Shred the meat off the breastbone and break the breastbone into two pieces. Reserve the meat and bones separately.

In a stockpot over medium-high heat, add the oil. Sauté the onion, carrot, celery, chicken wings, and breastbones for 8 to 10 minutes, or until vegetables soften.

Add the broth and water and stir to combine. Bring to a boil. Reduce the heat, cover, and simmer for 15 to 20 minutes, stirring occasionally. Add the noodles and cook for 5 minutes, stirring occasionally. Add reserved chicken and parsley and cook for 2 to 3 minutes. Discard the bones before serving. Season with salt and pepper.

PER SERVING

Calories	120
Fat	4 g
Saturated fat	1 g
Cholesterol	45 mg
Sodium	420 mg
Carbohydrate	5 g
Dietary fiber	1 g
Sugars	2 g
Protein	16 g
Calcium	30 mg
Potassium	210 mg

 TIP If your stomach is queasy, choose a rotisserie chicken with mild seasoning. Both traditional and lemon-pepper work well.

NOTES

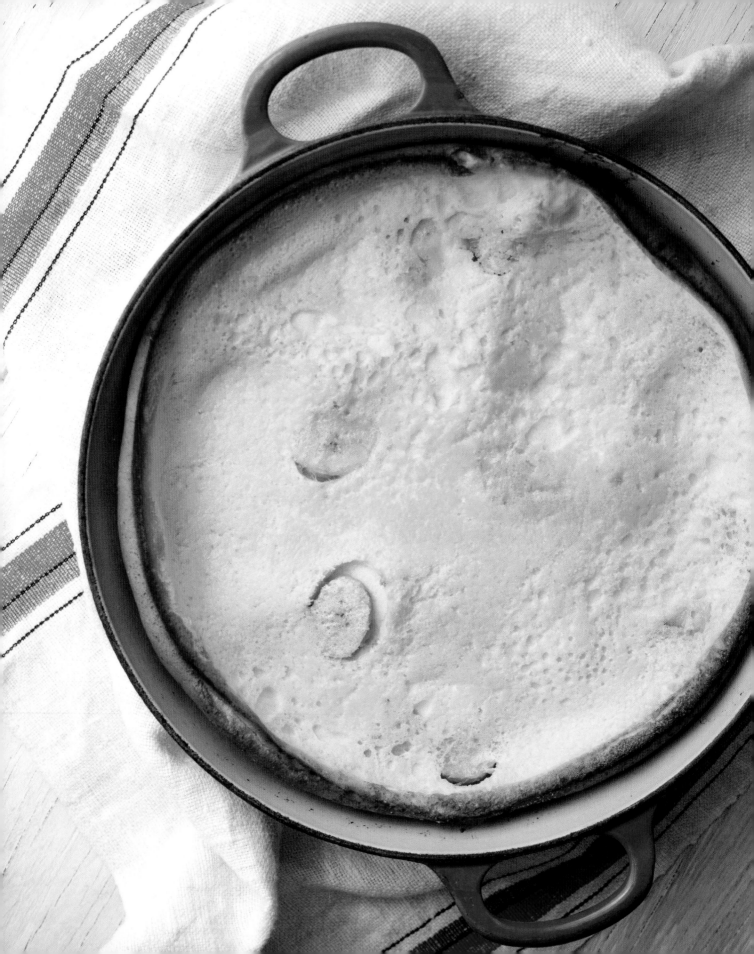

D DIARRHEA

Miso-Glazed Salmon

Chicken Congee

Rehydration Drinks

Fish in "Tomato Water"

Vegetable Broth

Baked Rice Balls

Lemon-Herb Tilapia Packets

Oatmeal-Banana-Peach Smoothie

Brown Sugar–Oatmeal Muffins

Banana Dutch Baby

Fruited Gelatin

Cran-Apple Slushie

Shrimp Dumplings with Dipping Sauce

Chicken and Aromatic Yellow Rice

Lemon Rice

Crispy Crunchy Fish Fingers

Citrus Tilapia

Mashed Potato–Chicken Patties

Herb-Flecked Popovers

YOU MAY EXPERIENCE DIARRHEA DURING TREATMENT. Diarrhea is the passage of loose or watery stools three or more times a day, with or without discomfort. Diarrhea can be caused by a number of factors during cancer treatment. Chemotherapy drugs, medications, and infection can all damage the normal, healthy cells that line the digestive tract. Surgery involving the stomach or intestines or radiation therapy to the abdomen or pelvis can alter the digestion and absorption of food and drink. In addition, if you are receiving more than one kind of treatment at the same time (such as radiation therapy and chemotherapy), your diarrhea could be worse. Diarrhea that is not controlled can lead to decreased strength and energy, poor appetite, dehydration, changes in blood pressure, and weight loss. Talk to your health care team for help managing your diarrhea.

There are several things you can do to lessen your diarrhea:

- Try to sip clear liquids throughout the day to prevent dehydration. Clear liquids are more than just water—see page 32 for what's allowed in a clear liquid diet.

- Room-temperature liquids may be easier to tolerate than cold or hot liquids. The majority of your liquids should be caffeine-free.

- Avoid greasy, fried, spicy, or very sweet foods, which can upset your stomach or irritate your intestines.

- Avoid high-fiber foods, such as whole grain breads and cereals and raw fruits and vegetables with the peel or skin left on. Gas-causing foods, such as dried beans and peas or cruciferous vegetables (like cabbage, cauliflower, broccoli, Brussels sprouts, etc.), can cause stomach upset even if they're cooked.

- Avoid sugar-free foods containing sorbitol, xylitol, or mannitol. They can worsen symptoms by making you gassy or bloated.

- Limit dairy products to no more than two cups per day—too much dairy can make symptoms worse.

When your diarrhea starts to improve, try the following suggestions:

- Small, more frequent meals may be easier on your system than larger meals.

- Begin eating small amounts of low-fiber, easy-to-digest foods, such as white rice, applesauce, bananas, mashed potatoes, dry white toast, pretzels, or plain crackers like oyster crackers or saltines.

- Replace sodium in your diet with soups, broths, sports drinks, oral rehydration solutions, pretzels, and plain crackers.

- Include foods that are high in potassium, such as bananas, potatoes without the skins, orange juice without the pulp, and sports drinks. Potassium is an important mineral that can be lost if you have diarrhea.

CONTACT YOUR DOCTOR IN THESE SITUATIONS:

- You have new or worsening abdominal pain or cramping.

- You have more than six watery stools in a 24-hour period with no improvement.

- Your stool has a strange color or odor or there is blood in your stool.

- You are taking anti-diarrhea medicine as directed and diarrhea is not stopping.

- You are unable to drink any liquids for more than two days.

For more information about managing diarrhea, visit the American Cancer Society website at cancer.org or call 800-227-2345.

LOW-FIBER FOODS

Dietary fiber is the indigestible part of plant foods. Low-fiber foods are often recommended if you are experiencing diarrhea. These foods are acceptable as part of a low-fiber diet:

Breads made from refined white flour or finely ground corn meal, such as English muffins, bagels, or white, potato, egg, or sourdough breads

Crackers, melba toast, and pretzels

Cereals such as corn flakes, Rice Krispies, or Rice or Corn Chex; hot cereals such as cream of wheat, cream of rice, instant oatmeal, and grits

Tender cuts of meat, poultry, or fish

Dairy (if tolerated), including milk, plain ice cream or ice milk, yogurt, sorbet, sherbet, and pudding

Cottage cheese, cream cheese, and mild hard cheeses such as American, Cheddar, and Monterey Jack

Eggs that are fully cooked or used in cooking

Creamy nut butters

Ripe bananas, avocado, and canned applesauce, peaches, pears

All vegetable juices (unless made from cruciferous vegetables such as broccoli, cabbage, cauliflower, and Brussels sprouts)

Tender, well-cooked vegetables such as green or wax beans, carrots, asparagus, mushrooms, beets, and winter and summer squash

Boiled, baked, or mashed potatoes (peeled)

Broth- or milk-based soups made with allowed vegetables (see above)

Miso-Glazed Salmon

A simple glaze made with soy sauce and miso (a Japanese paste made of fermented soybeans) is the perfect complement to baked salmon. Miso is found in the refrigerated section of most supermarkets.

When the salmon is almost done cooking, switch the oven setting from bake to broil to caramelize the sugar in the sauce. Keeping the baking pan in the middle position of the oven, away from the heating unit, prevents the topping from browning too quickly.

Apply the glaze before cooking and let it sit briefly to allow it to permeate the fish for greater flavor. Lining the pan with foil or parchment prevents sticking and speeds cleanup.

4 SERVINGS

2 tablespoons white miso paste

1 tablespoon mirin (Japanese rice wine)

1 tablespoon reduced-sodium soy sauce or tamari

1 tablespoon light brown sugar

1 tablespoon finely chopped fresh ginger

4 (4- to 6-ounce) salmon fillets

In a bowl, combine the miso, mirin, soy sauce, brown sugar, and ginger. Place the salmon skin side down in a baking pan and spread the miso mixture over it. Refrigerate for 30 to 60 minutes.

When ready to cook, place an oven rack in a middle setting. Preheat the oven to 400 degrees.

Bake for 10 to 14 minutes, or until cooked through. Change to the broil setting (keeping the baking pan in the middle setting) and broil for 1 to 3 minutes, or until the topping darkens and bubbles.

PER SERVING

Calories	190
Fat	9 g
Saturated fat	2 g
Cholesterol	60 mg
Sodium	300 mg
Carbohydrate	5 g
Dietary fiber	0 g
Sugars	3.5 g
Protein	23 g
Calcium	30 mg
Potassium	420 mg

TIP If you are experiencing neutropenia (see page 11), uncooked miso paste should be avoided.

Chicken Congee

Congee, also known as jook, is a soft, soupy rice dish, lightly seasoned with ginger and soy sauce for added appeal. If your stomach can handle it, add one large chicken breast at the beginning of cooking and simmer for twenty-five to thirty minutes, or until cooked through. Remove the chicken and let it cool before shredding the meat and adding it back during the last couple of minutes of cooking.

If you are experiencing taste changes and want more flavor, stir in a teaspoon or so of lime juice for acidity or fish sauce for saltiness and depth of flavor.

4 SERVINGS

6 cups homemade chicken broth (page 40) or store-bought reduced-sodium broth

1 (1-inch) piece fresh ginger, peeled and cut into 3 slices

1 teaspoon reduced-sodium soy sauce or tamari

2/3 cup basmati or jasmine rice, rinsed

In a stockpot, combine the broth, ginger, and soy sauce and bring to a boil. Reduce the heat and add the rice, stirring to combine. Simmer on low for 1 to 1 ½ hours, stirring occasionally, until the rice is very tender and much of the broth has been absorbed and the soup has thickened. Discard the ginger.

PER SERVING

Calories	130
Fat	1.5 g
Saturated fat	0 g
Cholesterol	10 mg
Sodium	790 mg
Carbohydrate	23 g
Dietary fiber	0 g
Sugars	0 g
Protein	6 g
Calcium	20 mg
Potassium	60 mg

 TIP If you want to add an easy-to-digest protein instead of (or in addition to) chicken, try adding eggs. Just before serving, beat two eggs and drizzle them into the simmering broth and stir to combine. The egg will cook quickly into fine threads.

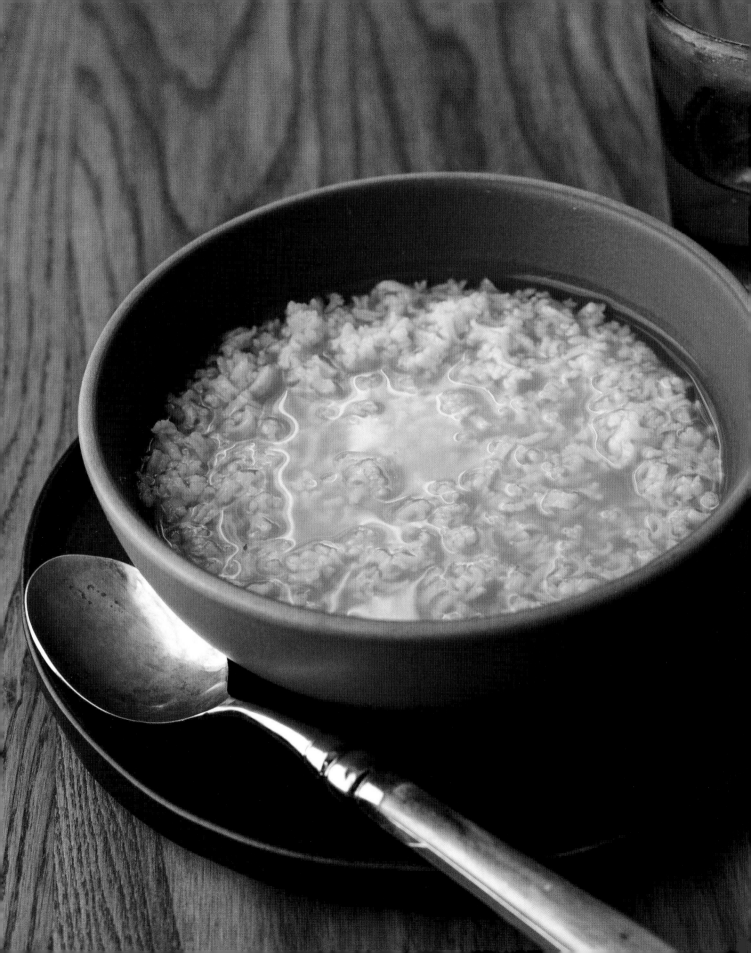

Rehydration Drinks

When you are experiencing diarrhea, keeping your body hydrated is key. Instead of spending money on expensive "sports drinks," keep these homemade drinks in your refrigerator to sip throughout the day. Small amounts of supplemental sugar contribute to their drinkability, and added salt provides needed electrolytes.

These drinks should be kept refrigerated and discarded after twenty-four hours.

Unflavored Rehydration Drink

For added flavor, add sliced citrus or Crystal Light powder to taste.

2 TO 4 SERVINGS

2 cups cold water

3 teaspoons granulated sugar

Heaping 1/4 teaspoon table salt

1/8 teaspoon baking soda

Lemon or lime slices or Crystal Light powder, optional

In a pitcher or closed container, combine the water, sugar, salt, and baking soda. Stir or shake well to combine. Add lemon, lime, or Crystal Light to taste, if desired. Keep refrigerated and stir again before pouring. Discard after 24 hours.

PER SERVING

Calories	25
Fat	0 g
Saturated fat	0 g
Cholesterol	0 mg
Sodium	470 mg
Carbohydrate	6 g
Dietary fiber	0 g
Sugars	6 g
Protein	0 g
Calcium	10 mg
Potassium	0 mg

Orange Rehydration Drink

This version adds orange juice to the mixture for more flavor.

2 TO 4 SERVINGS

2 cups cold water

½ cup freshly squeezed or 100 percent orange juice

4 teaspoons granulated sugar

¼ teaspoon table salt

⅛ teaspoon baking soda

In a pitcher or closed container, combine the water, orange juice, sugar, salt, and baking soda. Stir or shake well to combine. Keep refrigerated and stir before pouring. Discard after 24 hours.

PER SERVING

Calories	60
Fat	0 g
Saturated fat	0 g
Cholesterol	0 mg
Sodium	380 mg
Carbohydrate	15 g
Dietary fiber	0 g
Sugars	14 g
Protein	0 g
Calcium	10 mg
Potassium	120 mg

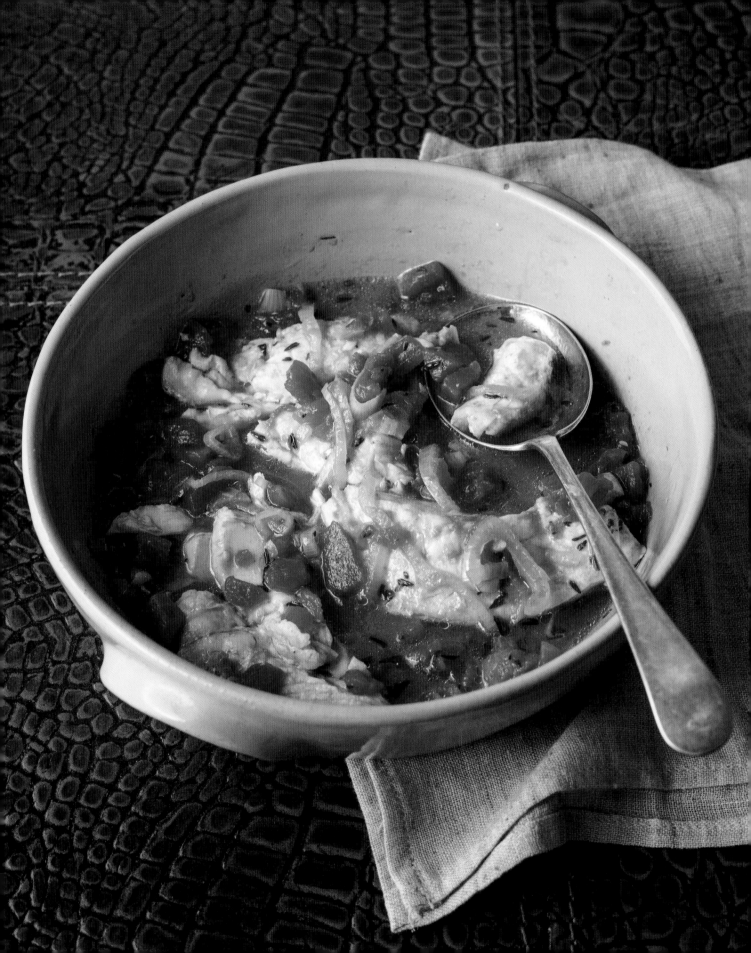

Fish in "Tomato Water"

Mild white fish fillets are poached in a light tomato and white wine broth for a meal that's easy on the stomach but doesn't feel depriving. Make sure you use a skillet with a tight-fitting lid.

Use canned petite cut tomatoes if you can find them. Or during the summer, substitute fresh, peeled, seeded tomatoes.

If you prefer not to cook with wine, just use water or broth and omit the wine.

4 SERVINGS

1 tablespoon olive oil

2 shallots, thinly sliced

1 cup white wine

¼ cup water

1 (14.5-ounce) can diced tomatoes

4 fresh thyme sprigs or ¼ teaspoon dried thyme

Salt and freshly ground black pepper

1 pound skinless white fish fillets, such as red snapper, halibut, or cod

In a large skillet over medium heat, add the oil. Add the shallots and sauté for 3 to 5 minutes, or until softened. Add the wine, water, tomatoes and their juice, and thyme and bring to a boil. Reduce the heat and simmer for 10 minutes, stirring occasionally. Season with salt and pepper. Add the fish in a single layer, spooning some of the broth over the fish to cover it. Cover and gently simmer for 7 to 10 minutes, or until the fish is cooked through. Discard the thyme sprigs.

PER SERVING

Calories	190
Fat	5 g
Saturated fat	1 g
Cholesterol	40 mg
Sodium	200 mg
Carbohydrate	7 g
Dietary fiber	1 g
Sugars	3 g
Protein	24 g
Calcium	70 mg
Potassium	710 mg

Vegetable Broth

Save extra veggie pieces and put them in a bag in the fridge or freezer to make your own vegetable broth. This combination delivers a broth with a pleasant, subtle flavor to drink on its own or to mix into soups. You can follow this exactly or use what you have on hand or see at the market. You can't go wrong with an approximate blend of these flavors. It's not necessary to peel the vegetables; just wash them well.

If it's hard to judge exactly how much the broth has reduced, look for a remnant liquid line on the sides of the pot, or for more accuracy, make a little mark on the side of the pot where the liquid starts to help gauge how much the broth has evaporated.

To coax out even more flavor, you can sauté the vegetables in a tablespoon or two of olive oil before adding the water, but this step isn't necessary.

5 SERVINGS

10 cups water

8 white mushrooms, coarsely chopped

2 celery stalks, coarsely chopped

2 large carrots, coarsely chopped

2 tomatoes, coarsely chopped

2 garlic cloves, smashed

1 medium onion, coarsely chopped

1 small fennel bulb, coarsely chopped

1 teaspoon salt

1 teaspoon black peppercorns

10 fresh Italian parsley sprigs

1 bay leaf

In a large stockpot, combine the water, mushrooms, celery, carrots, tomatoes, garlic, onion, fennel, salt, peppercorns, parsley, and bay leaf and bring to a boil. Reduce the heat and gently simmer for 1 to 1 ½ hours, or until the stock is reduced by about half. Set aside to cool briefly.

Place a large strainer in a large bowl or pot and carefully transfer the contents of the pot to the strainer, pushing down with a spoon to extract all the liquid. Discard the solids.

PER SERVING

Calories	5
Fat	0 g
Saturated fat	0 g
Cholesterol	0 mg
Sodium	410 mg
Carbohydrate	1 g
Dietary fiber	0 g
Sugars	0.5 g
Protein	0 g
Calcium	20 mg
Potassium	60 mg

 TIP Refrigerate until ready to use or eat. Freeze unused broth in quart containers to use later.

Baked Rice Balls

These mild baked nuggets of rice are simple enough to appeal even when you're feeling fragile. Adding Italian seasoning and using a stronger-flavored cheese, such as Parmesan, perks them up a little. For added flavor, family members can dip them in pasta sauce.

Make extra rice the night before to use for these balls.

15 BALLS

1 egg

1 ½ cups cooked white rice

½ cup grated or shredded mozzarella, Parmesan, or other cheese

2 tablespoons all-purpose flour

Salt and freshly ground black pepper

Pinch dried Italian seasoning, optional

1 cup pasta sauce, heated, optional

Preheat the oven to 350 degrees. Line a rimmed baking sheet with foil and lightly coat with nonstick cooking spray.

In a bowl, beat the egg. Add the rice, cheese, and flour and stir to combine. Sprinkle with salt, pepper, and Italian seasoning, if desired.

With wet hands, form the mixture into 1 ½-inch balls and place on the baking sheet. You may need to rewet your hands after every two to three balls.

Bake for 20 to 25 minutes, or until lightly golden. Serve with pasta sauce, if desired.

PER SERVING (ABOUT THREE BALLS)	
Calories	120
Fat	3 g
Saturated fat	1.5 g
Cholesterol	50 mg
Sodium	85 mg
Carbohydrate	16 g
Dietary fiber	0 g
Sugars	0 g
Protein	6 g
Calcium	100 mg
Potassium	40 mg

Lemon-Herb Tilapia Packets

The delicate flavors of fresh seafood, herbs, and citrus mingle pleasantly in this easy-to-prepare dish. Baking fish in these self-contained "packets" not only keeps it moist and succulent, it helps contain aromas for those who are sensitive to smells. If this is the case, open the packets in a different room from where you'll be eating.

Feel free to substitute another favorite fish—just adjust the cooking time because tilapia tends to be a thinner fillet, adding three to five minutes for thicker varieties, such as snapper or salmon.

Serve with white rice or plain pasta to absorb the sauce. For those not having diarrhea, serve with a favorite whole grain, such as brown rice, barley, or bulgur.

4 SERVINGS

4 (4- to 6-ounce) tilapia fillets

Salt and freshly ground black pepper

1 tablespoon finely chopped fresh dill

1 tablespoon finely chopped fresh Italian parsley

1 lemon, thinly sliced

¼ cup white wine

2 teaspoons extra virgin olive oil

Preheat the oven to 400 degrees.

Tear off four large pieces of foil or parchment paper. Place a piece of tilapia in the middle of each piece and sprinkle with salt and pepper. Top each fillet with dill and parsley and lay two to three lemon slices on top. Pull the sides of the foil up around the fish to make a "well." Drizzle each fillet with 1 tablespoon of wine and ½ teaspoon of olive oil. Fold the foil around the fish, pressing the edges to seal well. If using parchment, fold up the edges to seal. Place the packets on a baking sheet and bake for 10 to 14 minutes, or until cooked through.

To serve, place foil packs on individual plates and carefully open.

PER SERVING

Calories	140
Fat	4.5 g
Saturated fat	1 g
Cholesterol	50 mg
Sodium	50 mg
Carbohydrate	1 g
Dietary fiber	0 g
Sugars	0 g
Protein	22 g
Calcium	20 mg
Potassium	350 mg

TIP For the family (or when the side effect has resolved), add 1 tablespoon capers or sliced olives before baking for added flavor.

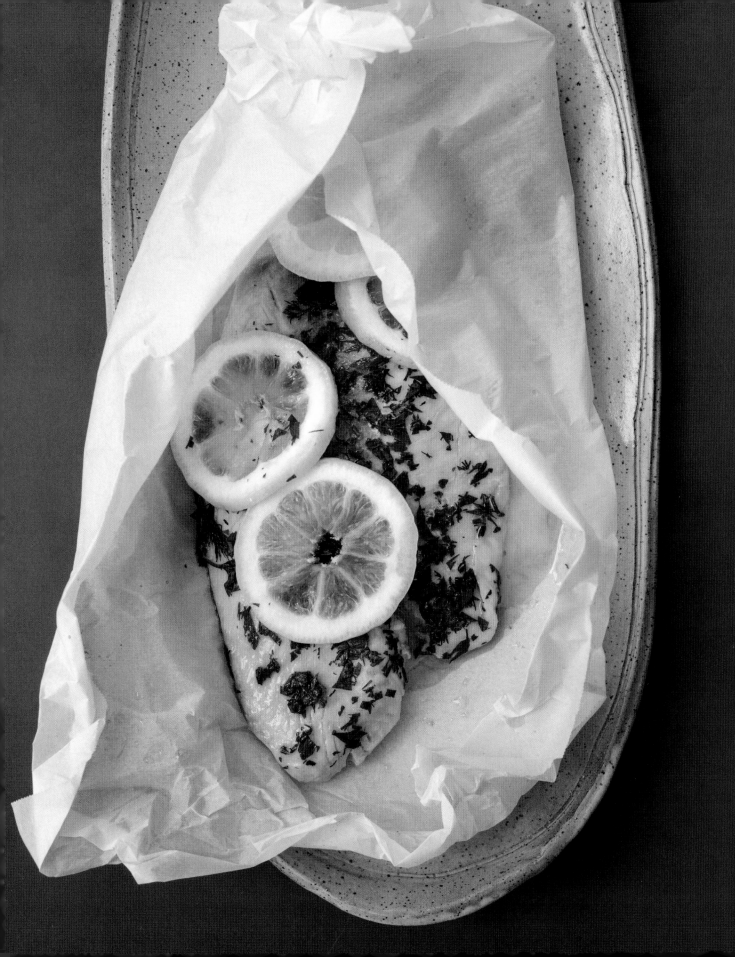

Oatmeal-Banana-Peach Smoothie

If you are having diarrhea, a shake fortified with water-soluble, fiber-filled oats will aid in the absorption of excess fluid in the bowel.

Bananas are also a good source of potassium and magnesium and are easily digested. Using probiotic yogurt and a plant-based milk instead of cow's milk can also help if you are sensitive to lactose. If you don't have yogurt on hand, just use the almond milk (or vice versa).

This recipe is also good for those having trouble swallowing because it makes a thicker shake than a regular smoothie. Start with one-half cup almond milk and add more to achieve the thickness you want.

2 SERVINGS

2 tablespoons old-fashioned rolled oats

½ to 1 cup almond milk

½ cup plain Greek yogurt

1 to 2 tablespoons honey

1 ripe banana, broken into pieces

1 cup frozen peaches

Pinch or 2 ground cinnamon

In a blender, purée the oats. Add ½ cup of the almond milk, yogurt, 1 tablespoon of the honey, banana, peaches, and cinnamon and blend until smooth. Taste and add more almond milk or honey, as desired.

PER SERVING

Calories	200
Fat	4 g
Saturated fat	1.5 g
Cholesterol	5 mg
Sodium	65 mg
Carbohydrate	37 g
Dietary fiber	4 g
Sugars	25 g
Protein	7 g
Calcium	180 mg
Potassium	540 mg

 TIP   Soy or cashew milk can be substituted for the almond milk, if you prefer.

Brown Sugar–Oatmeal Muffins

Heart-healthy oats give these mildly flavored muffins extra nutrients and provide binding action for those suffering from diarrhea. Soaking the oats in buttermilk helps soften them. For added flavor, increase the amount of cinnamon.

These muffins freeze well. Use just what you need and freeze the other muffins, defrosting one when you want something a little sweet.

12 MUFFINS

1 cup old-fashioned rolled oats

1 cup low-fat buttermilk

1 cup all-purpose flour

1 teaspoon baking powder

3/4 teaspoon ground cinnamon

1/2 teaspoon baking soda

1/2 teaspoon salt

2 eggs

1/2 cup packed light brown sugar

1/2 cup applesauce

1/3 cup canola oil

1 teaspoon vanilla extract

Preheat the oven to 400 degrees. Coat a muffin tin with nonstick cooking spray or fill with paper liners.

In a bowl, combine the oats and buttermilk. Set aside for 25 minutes.

Meanwhile, in a bowl, combine the flour, baking powder, cinnamon, baking soda, and salt.

In a separate bowl, beat the eggs. Add the brown sugar, applesauce, oil, and vanilla and stir to combine. Add to the oat mixture, stirring well to combine. Add the dry ingredients and stir gently to incorporate. Spoon the batter evenly into muffin cups.

Bake for 13 to 18 minutes, or until the tops just bounce back when touched. Leave in the tin for 5 minutes before transferring to a cooling rack.

PER SERVING
(ONE MUFFIN)

Calories	180
Fat	8 g
Saturated fat	1 g
Cholesterol	35 mg
Sodium	220 mg
Carbohydrate	25 g
Dietary fiber	1 g
Sugars	12 g
Protein	4 g
Calcium	70 mg
Potassium	120 mg

TIP With a few additions, these muffins are also a good option if you are experiencing constipation. Just add dried fruit, a chopped apple or pear, or nuts for additional fiber.

Banana Dutch Baby

Try this eggy, puffy pancake-like dish when you feel like treating yourself to an impressive-looking meal. Even though it takes just a few minutes to make and uses ingredients you probably have on hand, the batter rises so dramatically during baking that you feel a bit indulgent cutting into it.

If you don't feel like bananas, choose another low-fiber fruit, such as cooked apples or peaches. You can also skip the fruit and top it with seedless jam or powdered sugar if you feel like something sweeter.

For a savory Dutch baby, omit the sugar and vanilla and add a sprinkling of fresh herbs and/or shredded cheese.

Prepare the batter before preheating the oven to allow time for the flour to incorporate. The batter can also be made in a food processor.

4 SERVINGS

3 eggs

½ cup flour

½ cup milk

3 tablespoons granulated sugar, divided use

½ teaspoon vanilla extract

Pinch salt

2 tablespoons butter

1 banana, sliced

In a blender, combine the eggs, flour, milk, 2 tablespoons of the sugar, vanilla, and salt and process until smooth. Set aside while the oven heats.

Place a 10-inch skillet in the oven and preheat the oven to 425 degrees.

When the oven has preheated, carefully remove the hot skillet from the oven and add the butter, swirling it to evenly coat the inside surface. Place the banana slices on the bottom of the skillet and sprinkle with the remaining 1 tablespoon of sugar.

Re-whisk the batter and pour it into the hot skillet. Don't be concerned if the butter rises to the edges around the batter.

Bake for 18 to 20 minutes, or until the edges begin to form a dark golden brown crust.

PER SERVING

Calories	250
Fat	11 g
Saturated fat	5 g
Cholesterol	160 mg
Sodium	150 mg
Carbohydrate	30 g
Dietary fiber	1 g
Sugars	15 g
Protein	8 g
Calcium	60 mg
Potassium	220 mg

 TIP To allow the batter to rise fully, do not open the oven during cooking.

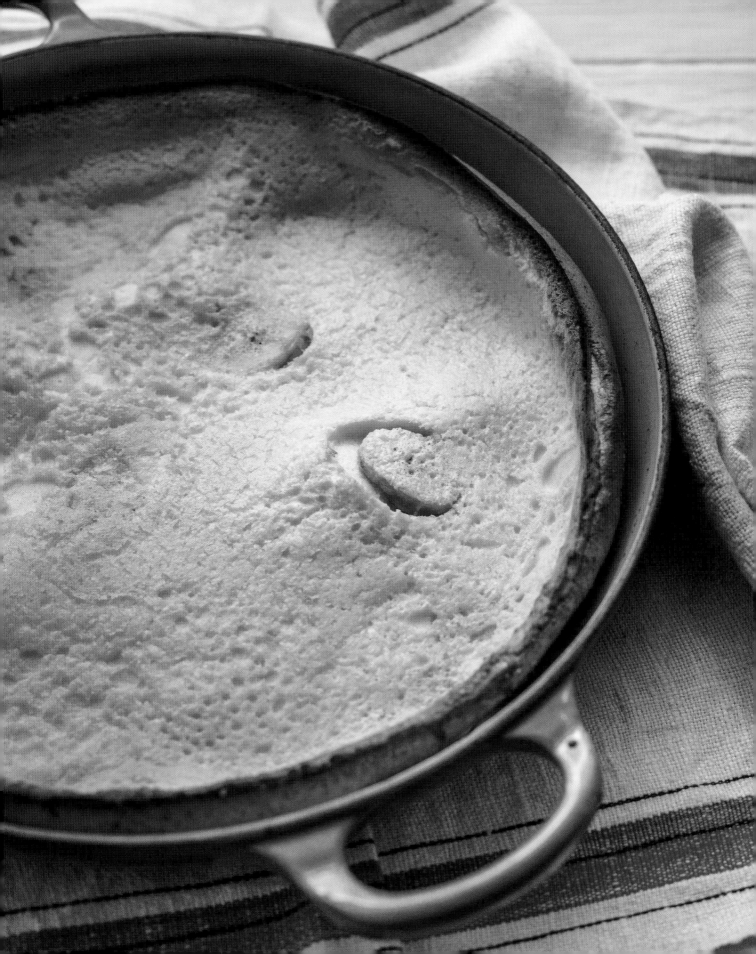

Fruited Gelatin

For delicate stomachs and sensitive mouths, a gelatin mold fits the bill, providing hydration and calories until symptoms resolve. Don't use apple juice or tropical fruit mix—they could aggravate diarrhea.

8 SERVINGS

2 (3-ounce, 4-serving) boxes flavored gelatin

2 cups boiling water

1 (15-ounce) can mixed fruit in 100 percent juice

3/4 to 1 cup 100 percent white grape juice or grape juice, chilled

In a heat-proof bowl, stir the gelatin powder and boiling water until completely dissolved.

Drain canned fruit juice into a measuring cup, reserving fruit. Add enough of the grape juice to make 1 ¼ cups. Stir juice into the gelatin mixture and refrigerate for about 2 hours, or until slightly thickened.

Add the reserved fruit and stir gently to incorporate. Pour into a lightly greased 4- to 6-cup mold. Refrigerate for 3 to 4 hours, or until firm.

PER SERVING	
Calories	130
Fat	0 g
Saturated fat	0 g
Cholesterol	0 mg
Sodium	85 mg
Carbohydrate	30 g
Dietary fiber	0.5 g
Sugars	28 g
Protein	1 g
Calcium	10 mg
Potassium	80 mg

 TIP If you have diabetes, consider using sugar-free gelatin.

Cran-Apple Slushie

Whenever you find yourself with extra fruit juice that you won't use for a while, pour it into an ice cube tray and freeze it to use later. Large amounts of apple juice can aggravate diarrhea, but in small amounts, it is typically tolerated.

In this combination, frozen apple juice is blended with cranberry juice for a cran-apple slushie to sip for hydration when you don't feel up to eating. Customize the flavor by using whichever fruit juices you enjoy.

1 SERVING

1/2 cup 100 percent apple juice

1/2 cup 100 percent cranberry juice, chilled

Pour apple juice into an ice cube tray and freeze for 2 or more hours, or until solid.

In a blender, combine the cranberry juice and apple juice ice cubes and blend until frothy. Drink immediately.

PER SERVING

Calories	115
Fat	0 g
Saturated fat	0 g
Cholesterol	0 mg
Sodium	5 mg
Carbohydrate	29 g
Dietary fiber	0 g
Sugars	27 g
Protein	0.5 g
Calcium	20 mg
Potassium	220 mg

 TIP Most standard ice-cube trays hold about 1 cup of liquid. Measure your tray's capacity to know how many cubes a half-cup of juice makes.

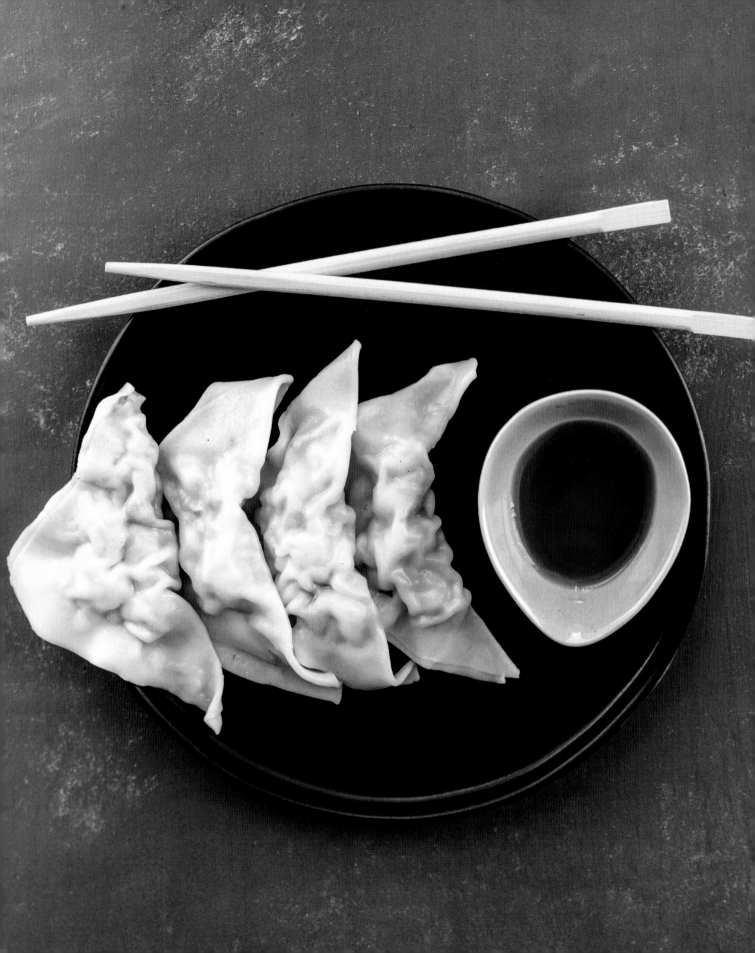

Shrimp Dumplings with Dipping Sauce

Don't be intimidated by the thought of making your own dumplings. With premade wrappers, these delicate filled treats come together quickly.

Serve the dipping sauce on the side for dunking or drizzle the dumplings with sauce before eating.

Experiment with other fillings—ground chicken is another good option.

20 DUMPLINGS

DIPPING SAUCE:

¼ cup reduced-sodium soy sauce or tamari

¼ cup unseasoned rice vinegar

1 tablespoon honey

1 teaspoon sesame oil

DUMPLINGS:

8 ounces peeled uncooked shrimp, chopped

1 finely chopped scallion

1 tablespoon finely chopped fresh cilantro

2 teaspoons minced fresh ginger

1 teaspoon reduced-sodium soy sauce or tamari

1 egg white

1 tablespoon cold water

20 dumpling, wonton, or gyoza wrappers

Prepare the dipping sauce: In a bowl, combine the soy sauce, rice vinegar, honey, and sesame oil. Set aside.

In a bowl, combine the shrimp, scallion, cilantro, ginger, and soy sauce.

In a bowl, combine the egg white and water.

Working in batches, line up dumpling wrappers on a work surface. Brush the egg wash over the wrapper and place 1 teaspoon of filling in the center of each wrapper. Fold the wrapper in half and pinch the edges to seal the dumpling. Repeat with remaining filling and wrappers.

Fill a stockpot two-thirds full with water and bring to a boil. Reduce the heat to a simmer and drop in dumplings, eight to ten at a time. After they rise to the surface, simmer for 4 minutes, then remove with a slotted spoon. Repeat with remaining dumplings.

Serve with the dipping sauce.

PER SERVING
(ONE DUMPLING)

Calories	40
Fat	0 g
Saturated fat	0 g
Cholesterol	15 mg
Sodium	150 mg
Carbohydrate	6 g
Dietary fiber	0 g
Sugars	1 g
Protein	3 g
Calcium	10 mg
Potassium	40 mg

Chicken and Aromatic Yellow Rice

This chicken and rice combination made with gentle seasonings that aid digestion is a welcome meal when you are having intestinal distress. Even better, it all cooks in one pot, making cleanup a breeze.

Star anise is a flower-shaped seed with a gentle licorice flavor and is used frequently in Chinese and Indian cuisine. Cardamom, a light green pod with seeds inside, is a member of the ginger family and is also frequently used in Indian cuisine.

4 SERVINGS

1 pound boneless, skinless chicken breasts, cut into 3/4-inch pieces

Salt and freshly ground black pepper

2 tablespoons olive oil, divided use

1/2 small onion, finely chopped

5 crushed cardamom pods

3 star anise

1 teaspoon ground turmeric

1 cup basmati rice, rinsed

1 1/2 cups homemade chicken broth (page 40) or store-bought reduced-sodium broth

Sprinkle the chicken with salt and pepper.

In a large skillet over medium-high heat, add 1 tablespoon of the oil. Cook the chicken for 2 to 3 minutes per side, or until lightly golden brown and cooked through. Remove the chicken and set aside.

In the same skillet, add the remaining 1 tablespoon of oil. Sauté the onion for 3 to 5 minutes, or until softened. Add the cardamom pods, star anise, and turmeric and stir to combine. Add the rice and sauté for 1 minute. Add the broth and bring to a boil, stirring frequently to dislodge any bits of food that might have stuck to the bottom of the skillet. Reduce the heat to low, cover, and cook for 12 to 15 minutes, or until the liquid has been absorbed. Discard the cardamom pods and star anise. Return the chicken to the skillet and stir to combine. Cover and cook for 1 to 2 minutes, or until the chicken is heated through. Season with salt and pepper.

PER SERVING	
Calories	360
Fat	10 g
Saturated fat	2 g
Cholesterol	65 mg
Sodium	250 mg
Carbohydrate	35 g
Dietary fiber	1 g
Sugars	0.5 g
Protein	28 g
Calcium	30 mg
Potassium	290 mg

TIP For the family (or when the side effect has resolved), mix in a half-cup or more of dried fruit, such as chopped apricots, dried cranberries, currants, and/or raisins before serving for fiber and flavor. Top with slivered almonds for added crunch.

Lemon Rice

This gently flavored rice provides a little variety when you are being cautious about food selection. Its subtle notes of citrus pair well with Fish in "Tomato Water" (page 73) or the Miso-Glazed Salmon (page 67).

If using basmati or jasmine rice, rinse it before cooking.

4 SERVINGS

2 teaspoons butter

1 cup basmati, jasmine, or other white rice

¼ teaspoon ground turmeric

1 ¾ cups homemade chicken broth (page 40) or store-bought reduced-sodium broth

1 lemon, zested and juiced

Salt and freshly ground black pepper

In a saucepan over medium heat, melt the butter. Add the rice and turmeric and stir to combine. Add the broth, 3 tablespoons of the lemon juice, and the lemon zest. Bring to a boil, reduce the heat, cover, and simmer for 15 to 20 minutes, or until the broth is absorbed. Season with salt and pepper and additional lemon juice, if desired.

PER SERVING	
Calories	180
Fat	2.5 g
Saturated fat	1.5 g
Cholesterol	10 mg
Sodium	240 mg
Carbohydrate	35 g
Dietary fiber	1 g
Sugars	0 g
Protein	4 g
Calcium	20 mg
Potassium	80 mg

Crispy Crunchy Fish Fingers

When you favor milder flavors, adding a crispy texture can help make food more interesting. Panko is lower in fiber than regular bread crumbs, but it is coarser so it provides more crunch.

Line the baking sheets with foil or parchment paper to make cleanup a breeze.

4 SERVINGS

1 pound cod fillets, cut into 1-inch "strips"

1 cup buttermilk

1 tablespoon olive oil

1/2 cup cornstarch

1 egg

1 cup panko

1/2 teaspoon salt

1/2 teaspoon fresh thyme leaves or 1/4 teaspoon dried thyme

1/4 teaspoon garlic powder

In a bowl, combine the fish and buttermilk. Refrigerate for 20 to 30 minutes.

When ready to cook, preheat the oven to 425 degrees. With a brush or spatula, spread the oil on a baking sheet.

Place the cornstarch on a plate. In a shallow bowl, beat the egg. On a separate plate, combine the panko, salt, thyme, and garlic powder.

Remove the fish from the buttermilk, letting any excess drip off. Coat the fish in the cornstarch, then dip in the egg, letting any excess drip off. Coat with the panko mixture, pressing to adhere.

Place the fish on the baking sheet and bake for 12 to 15 minutes, flipping the fish after 8 minutes.

PER SERVING

Calories	280
Fat	6 g
Saturated fat	1 g
Cholesterol	95 mg
Sodium	410 mg
Carbohydrate	29 g
Dietary fiber	2 g
Sugars	1 g
Protein	25 g
Calcium	70 mg
Potassium	290 mg

TIP For the family (or when the side effect has resolved), serve with tartar sauce or try a homemade yogurt-honey mustard dipping sauce: combine 1/2 cup plain Greek yogurt with 2 tablespoons Dijon or whole grain mustard and 2 tablespoons honey.

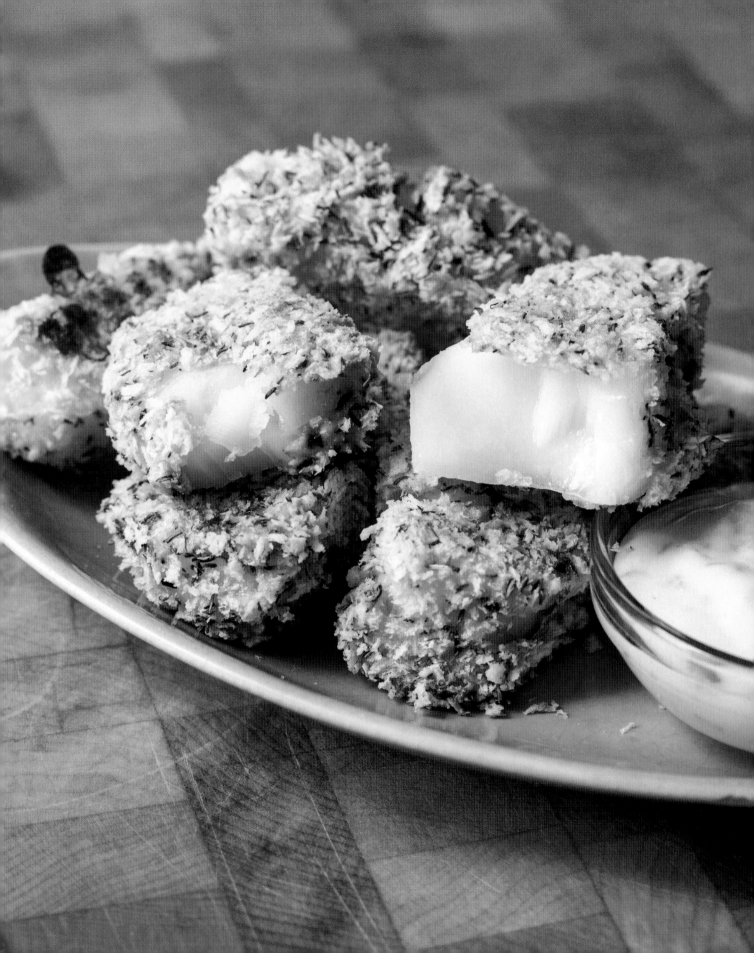

Citrus Tilapia

This light fish entrée gets a flavor boost from a citrus glaze made from fresh lemon juice, orange juice, and fresh ginger. For stronger, more acidic flavor, add lemon zest and additional juice. Make sure to use a high-quality 100 percent orange juice that is freshly squeezed (not from concentrate).

4 SERVINGS

2 tablespoons all-purpose flour

Salt and freshly ground black pepper

1 pound tilapia fillets

1 tablespoon olive oil

1 tablespoon butter

½ cup freshly squeezed or 100 percent orange juice

1 lemon, zested and juiced

½ teaspoon grated fresh ginger

On a plate, combine the flour and a sprinkle of salt and pepper. Lightly dredge the tilapia in the flour.

In a large skillet over medium heat, add the oil and butter. When the butter has melted, add the fish and cook for 2 to 3 minutes per side, or until golden and just cooked through. Remove the fish and set aside.

Add the orange juice, 2 tablespoons of the lemon juice, and the ginger to the skillet. Increase the heat and simmer for 1 to 2 minutes, or until thickened, stirring occasionally. Taste and add lemon zest or more lemon juice if necessary. Return the fish to the skillet, coat with sauce, and cook for 1 to 2 minutes, or until heated through.

PER SERVING	
Calories	200
Fat	9 g
Saturated fat	3.5 g
Cholesterol	80 mg
Sodium	55 mg
Carbohydrate	7 g
Dietary fiber	0 g
Sugars	3 g
Protein	23 g
Calcium	10 mg
Potassium	440 mg

Mashed Potato–Chicken Patties

These little patties are perfect for sensitive stomachs and for those looking for an easy-to-eat small meal. Each bite provides comfort and sustenance. Cooked chicken breast adds lean protein while the potatoes provide carbohydrates.

This combination is also a great way to use up the leftovers from a chicken and potato dinner. Use a food processor to grind the chicken quickly.

8 SERVINGS

¼ cup all-purpose flour

Salt and freshly ground black pepper

1 egg

1 cup cooled mashed potatoes

1 cup (about 4 ounces) cooked ground or very finely chopped chicken breast

1 tablespoon canola oil

On a plate, combine the flour and a sprinkle of salt and pepper.

In a bowl, beat the egg. Add the mashed potatoes and chicken. Form the mixture into 2-inch balls. Lightly dredge the balls in the flour. You may need to wet your hands after every 3 to 4 balls.

In a large, preferably nonstick, skillet over medium heat, add the oil. Add the balls and flatten into patties with a spatula (they should be about 2 ½ inches wide). Cook for 5 to 8 minutes per side, or until crispy and golden.

PER SERVING
(ONE PATTY)

Calories	90
Fat	4 g
Saturated fat	1 g
Cholesterol	40 mg
Sodium	85 mg
Carbohydrate	7 g
Dietary fiber	0 g
Sugars	0 g
Protein	6 g
Calcium	10 mg
Potassium	120 mg

TIP If you don't have leftover mashed potatoes, make your own or buy refrigerated premade mashed potatoes. For a time-saving dinner, use leftover rotisserie chicken and finely chop.

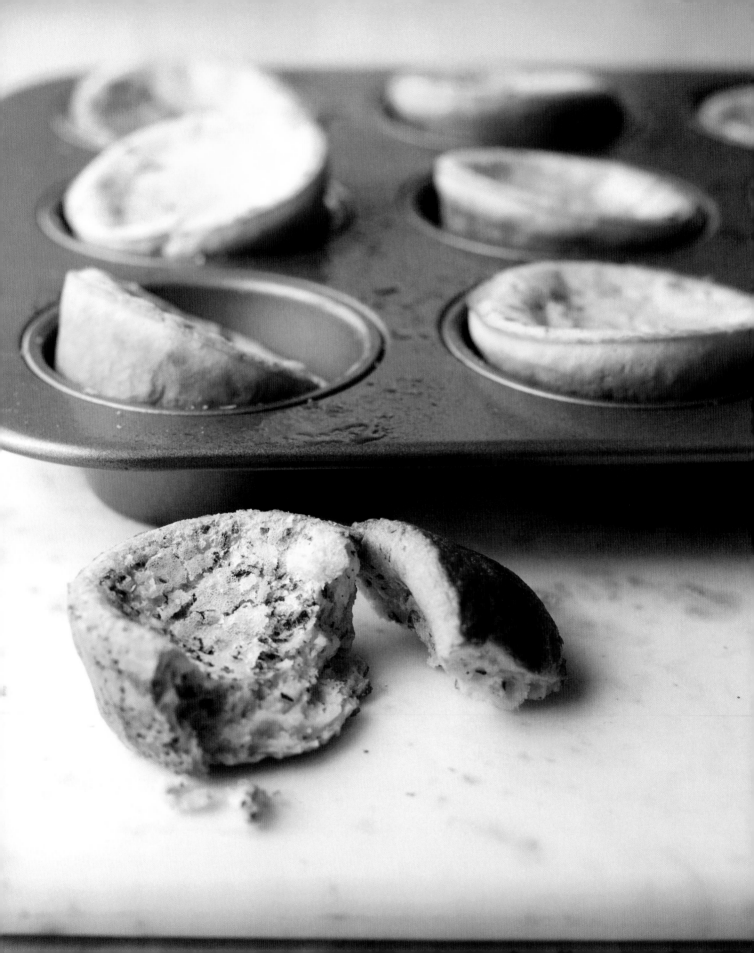

Herb-Flecked Popovers

When your stomach is queasy, there's no need to limit yourself to dry crackers. For something different but still comforting to nibble on, try a crispy popover. As "fancy" as they seem, popovers take less than five minutes to make using a blender. The top-hat shape comes from steam forming inside them while they bake, literally making the batter pop over the edges of the pan. The result is a soft texture inside and a crunchy exterior.

Give the baking tin a good coating of nonstick cooking spray, butter, or oil to prevent sticking. As tempting as it is, don't open the oven door as they bake or the popovers could flatten.

The fresh herbs add subtle flavor, but the popovers are equally good without.

8 TO 10 SERVINGS

1 cup milk

1 cup all-purpose flour

2 eggs

1/2 teaspoon salt

1 tablespoon butter, melted

2 tablespoons finely chopped assorted fresh herbs, such as Italian parsley, basil, chives, dill, and thyme

Preheat the oven to 400 degrees. Generously coat a muffin tin with nonstick cooking spray.

In a blender, combine the milk, flour, eggs, salt, and butter. Process until smooth, scraping down the sides if necessary. Add the herbs and pulse to combine. Fill the muffin cups one-half to two-thirds full with batter and place in the center of the oven. Bake for 25 to 35 minutes, or until puffed, golden brown, and crisp.

PER SERVING

Calories	100
Fat	3 g
Saturated fat	1 g
Cholesterol	50 mg
Sodium	190 mg
Carbohydrate	14 g
Dietary fiber	0 g
Sugars	2 g
Protein	4 g
Calcium	50 mg
Potassium	80 mg

 TIP For a plain popover, omit the herbs.

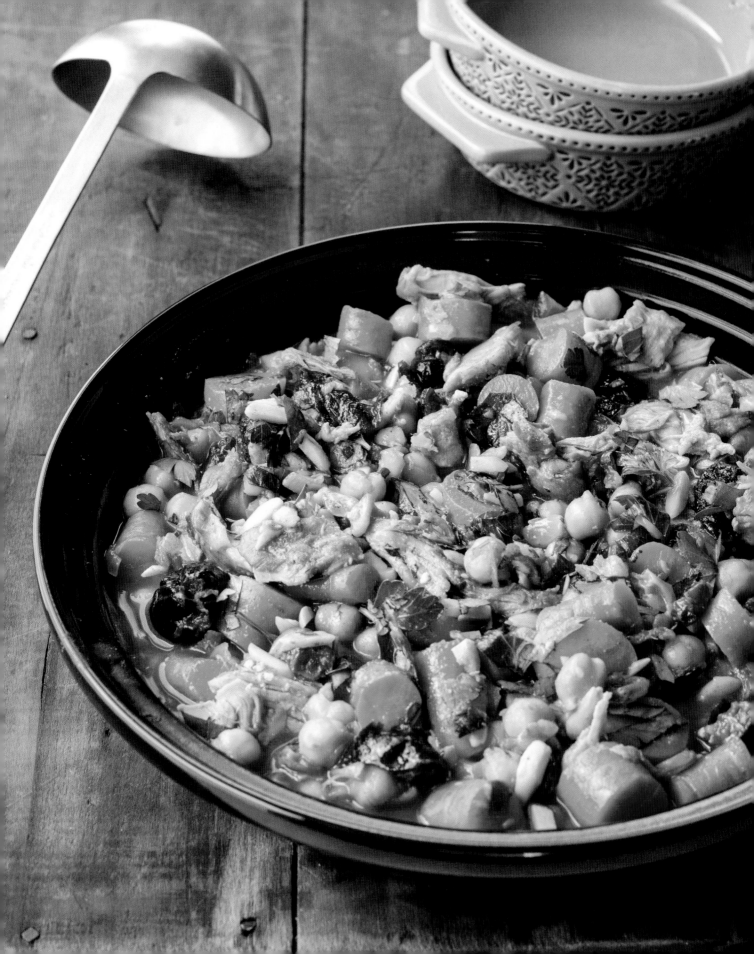

C CONSTIPATION

Tandoori Turkey Kebabs with Herb Salad

Super-Veggie Fried Rice

Socca (Chickpea Flatbread)

Chicken Tagine with Carrots, Prunes, and Chickpeas

Whole Grain Penne with Roasted Eggplant and Tomatoes

Vegetable, Lentil, and Farro St-oup

Date and Fruit Bread

Spinach and Brown Rice "Pie"

Bulgur Salad with Dried Fruit

Fig, Apple, and Apricot Compote

Date Jam

Multigrain Almond Butter and Date Jam Sandwich

Crunchy Roasted Lemon-Garlic Chickpeas

Fiber-Filled Trail Mix

Honey-Bran Muffins

Raspberry Chia Pudding

Granola with Almond, Apples, and Ginger

Tuna Salad

Baked Sweet Potato and Beet Chips

CONSTIPATION IS A COMMON CONCERN DURING CANCER TREATMENT. Constipation is being unable to move your bowels as often or having to push harder to have a bowel movement. Constipation can make you uncomfortable, and you may not feel like eating and drinking. If you are constipated, you may also experience abdominal discomfort or pain from cramping, bloating, gas, and hard stools.

Constipation can be caused by medications, both for cancer and for pain. Some chemotherapy treatments or some anti-nausea medications can also be constipating. Constipation may also occur if you have been asked to take vitamin and mineral supplements such as iron or calcium. You are at risk for constipation if you are less active, not drinking enough fluid, or if you are eating a low-fiber diet. It is important to keep your bowel movements regular and easy to pass.

To help prevent and manage constipation during your cancer treatment, try the following suggestions:

- Try to drink eight cups of liquids each day, unless otherwise directed by your health care team. Good options are water, fruit and vegetable juices, fruit nectars, sports drinks, gelatin, popsicles, ices, sherbet, broth, and bouillon.

- Drink warm or hot liquids. Try warm prune juice, decaffeinated tea or coffee, or hot water with lemon juice and honey. Avoid drinking too many liquids that contain caffeine.

- Get as much light exercise as possible. Physical activity can help stimulate your bowels. Talk to your health care team about what types of activity are best for you.

Try making changes in your diet to help soften your stool and stimulate bowel function:

- Eat meals and snacks at regular times each day.

- Add high-fiber foods:

   Raw or cooked fruits and vegetables with the skin and peel on (unless otherwise directed by your health care team)

   100 percent bran or whole grain foods such as cereals, bread, popcorn, brown rice, or whole wheat pasta

   Beans, peas, seeds, and nuts

   Dried fruit such as apricots, prunes, raisins, apples, figs, and dates

HIGH-FIBER FOODS

Dietary fiber, also known as roughage, is the indigestible part of a plant. There are two types of fiber in foods, and both should be increased if you are constipated. *Soluble fiber* helps to bind water in the stool, softening the stool. Foods that contain soluble fiber include oat bran, bananas, applesauce, potatoes, cornmeal, oats, and rice. *Insoluble fiber* should be increased when you have constipation to help stimulate the bowels to move. Insoluble fiber can be found in the peel and skin of vegetables and fruits, and in whole grains, seeds, and nuts.

High-fiber foods include plant foods such as fresh or dried fruits, vegetables, whole grains, nuts, seeds, popcorn, wheat or oat bran, and legumes (dried beans and peas). In general, it is best to get fiber from foods rather than supplements. Sometimes, however, your dietitian or doctor may recommend that you take a fiber supplement, such as Benefiber, Metamucil, Citracel, or FiberCon. Check with your health care team before starting fiber supplements or if you have questions about fiber.

- Experts advise eating twenty-five to thirty-five grams of dietary fiber each day. The right amount of fiber can be different for each person, depending on your needs and your ability to digest it.

- Talk to a registered dietitian about what to eat if you are constipated.

If you are bloated or having problems with gas, avoid these gas-producing foods and beverages:

- Beans, peas, and nuts

- Vegetables such as broccoli, cauliflower, Brussels sprouts, cabbage, onions, garlic, cucumber, and bell peppers

- Carbonated beverages

To lessen the amount of air you swallow while eating, try not to talk much at meals, avoid drinking with straws, and avoid chewing gum.

If you are at risk for or have constipation, seek help from your health care team to set up a daily bowel care plan that is best for you. To help keep your bowel movements regular, your health care team may advise you to take over-the-counter products, such as fiber supplements, stool softeners, and gentle stimulants. Be sure to ask your health care team what products are right for you, and use laxatives or enemas only with the advice of your health care team.

CONTACT YOUR DOCTOR IN THESE SITUATIONS:

- You have blood in or around the anal area or in your stool.

- You are having persistent abdominal cramping or vomiting.

- You have had fewer than three bowel movements in one week.

For more information about managing constipation, visit the American Cancer Society website at cancer.org or call 800-227-2345.

NOTES

PER SERVING

Calories	220
Fat	6 g
Saturated fat	1.5 g
Cholesterol	70 mg
Sodium	250 mg
Carbohydrate	11 g
Dietary fiber	3 g
Sugars	1 g
Protein	29 g
Calcium	60 mg
Potassium	390 mg

Tandoori Turkey Kebabs with Herb Salad

For variety, turkey replaces chicken in these kebabs. In addition to its probiotic qualities, a yogurt marinade has tenderizing properties. If you don't feel up to the bulgur salad, enjoy the kebabs on their own.

Prepare the herb salad before skewering the turkey and preheating the oven, or if time allows, make it ahead and refrigerate so that the flavors have time to meld. If you don't have time to make the herb salad, serve with tzatziki sauce.

If you don't have metal skewers, place wooden ones in water for an hour to minimize burning.

4 SERVINGS

2 garlic cloves

1 (1-inch) piece fresh ginger, peeled and coarsely chopped

1/2 onion, quartered

1 (6-ounce) container or 3/4 cup plain or Greek yogurt

2 teaspoons ground cumin

1 teaspoon salt

1/2 teaspoon ground turmeric

1 pound boneless, skinless turkey breast, cut in 1-inch pieces

1/4 cup bulgur

1/4 to 1/3 cup boiling water

1 cup chopped fresh Italian parsley

1 cup chopped assorted fresh herbs, such as basil, chives, dill, and mint

1 small cucumber, seeded and chopped

1 lemon, zested and juiced

1 tablespoon extra-virgin olive oil

Salt and freshly ground black pepper

In a food processor, pulse the garlic, ginger, and onion until coarsely chopped. Add the yogurt, cumin, salt, and turmeric and pulse to combine, scraping down the blade and sides to blend. Transfer to a bowl or zip-top bag and add the turkey to the marinade, turning to coat the pieces. Refrigerate for 4 to 24 hours.

In a heatproof bowl, combine the bulgur and 1/4 cup of the water. Set aside for 30 minutes (if mixture absorbs the water too quickly, add 1 or more tablespoons hot water until absorbed and the bulgur is tender). Add the parsley, assorted herbs, cucumber, lemon zest, 2 tablespoons of the lemon juice, and olive oil. Taste and add more lemon juice, if desired. Season with salt and pepper.

When ready to cook, place one oven rack in the top position and the other in a middle slot. Preheat the oven to 400 degrees.

Remove the turkey from the marinade, letting any excess drip off, and thread on skewers. Place the skewers on a rimmed baking sheet.

Bake for 20 to 25 minutes, or until cooked through. Change to the broil setting and transfer the baking sheet to the top shelf and broil for 30 to 60 seconds, rotating the skewers for added browning.

Super-Veggie Fried Rice

This version of a take-out standard is given a healthy twist by substituting brown rice for white and loading it up with vegetables. The dynamic duo of frozen peas and carrots is used for convenience, but throw in any extra veggies you have in the fridge. Brown rice freezes well; when you make plain brown rice as a side dish, cook an extra couple of cups to freeze for future use. Then when you're craving something salty, savory, and high in fiber, you'll have everything you need to put this dish together quickly.

4 SERVINGS

2 eggs

1 to 2 tablespoons reduced-sodium soy sauce or tamari

1 tablespoon canola oil

2 scallions, thinly sliced

2 garlic cloves, minced

1 tablespoon finely chopped fresh ginger

1 cup frozen peas and carrots

1 cup frozen chopped broccoli

2 cups cooked brown rice

In a bowl, beat the eggs and 1 tablespoon of the soy sauce. Set aside.

In a large skillet over medium-high heat, add the oil. Add the scallions, garlic, and ginger and sauté for 1 minute. Add the peas and carrots and broccoli and sauté until heated through. Add the rice and sauté until heated through. Move the rice mixture to the side and add the eggs to the empty space in the skillet. Cook until just set, then mix to scramble. Stir to combine with the rice. Taste and add a few shakes of soy sauce, if desired.

PER SERVING

Calories	230
Fat	7 g
Saturated fat	1.5 g
Cholesterol	90 mg
Sodium	220 mg
Carbohydrate	32 g
Dietary fiber	4 g
Sugars	3 g
Protein	9 g
Calcium	50 mg
Potassium	290 mg

TIP Add toasted sesame seeds or almonds for extra crunch and fiber. For extra protein, add tofu or cooked chicken or shrimp.

Socca (Chickpea Flatbread)

This skillet-baked flatbread, known as socca in France and farinata in Italy, uses chickpea flour, which is gluten-free and rich in protein and fiber. Eat warm straight from the skillet as is, or top with a light coating of yogurt or hummus and add lightly dressed greens or roasted vegetables for a heartier pizza-like meal.

Let the batter rest, covered, for at least two and up to twelve hours in the refrigerator, to allow the flour to absorb the water.

4 SERVINGS

1 cup chickpea flour

1 teaspoon salt

1 cup lukewarm water

3 tablespoons olive oil, divided use

1 teaspoon finely chopped fresh rosemary, optional

In a bowl, combine the chickpea flour and salt. Gradually whisk in the water and 1 tablespoon of the olive oil. Cover and refrigerate for 2 or more hours. A film will form on top of the batter; scrape off before using.

When ready to cook, set an oven rack in the second-closest setting to the broiler and place a 12-inch skillet in the oven. Preheat the oven to 450 degrees.

Carefully remove the hot skillet from the oven and add the remaining 2 tablespoons of olive oil, swirling it to evenly coat the inside surface.

Rewhisk the batter and add the rosemary, if desired. Pour the batter into the hot skillet. Don't be concerned if the oil rises to the surface around the batter.

Bake for 6 to 8 minutes, or until the edges begin to form a crust. Change to the broil setting and cook for 1 to 2 minutes, or until the top begins to brown in spots.

Remove the skillet from the oven and use a spatula to transfer the flatbread to a cutting board. Slice into wedges and/or top with additional ingredients, if desired.

PER SERVING

Calories	180
Fat	12 g
Saturated fat	1.5 g
Cholesterol	0 mg
Sodium	600 mg
Carbohydrate	13 g
Dietary fiber	3 g
Sugars	3 g
Protein	5 g
Calcium	10 mg
Potassium	200 mg

Chicken Tagine with Carrots, Prunes, and Chickpeas

This fiber-full dish features chicken thighs nestled alongside carrots, dried fruit, and chickpeas and seasoned with the warming flavors of a Moroccan-inspired spice blend. Serve it over quinoa or brown rice for added nutrients and fiber.

4 SERVINGS

1 1/2 pounds boneless, skinless chicken thighs, trimmed of excess fat

Salt and freshly ground black pepper

1 tablespoon olive oil

1 onion, chopped

3 garlic cloves, minced

1 teaspoon ground coriander

1 teaspoon ground cinnamon

1 teaspoon ground cumin

1/2 teaspoon paprika

1/2 teaspoon ground ginger

2 cups homemade chicken broth (page 40) or store-bought reduced-sodium broth

10 pitted prunes, cut in half

5 carrots, cut into 1-inch pieces

1 cup canned chickpeas, rinsed and drained

1/3 cup raisins, golden raisins, or chopped apricots

1/2 cup slivered almonds, toasted

1/4 cup chopped fresh Italian parsley or cilantro, optional

Sprinkle the chicken with salt and pepper.

In a large skillet over medium-high heat, add the oil. Cook the chicken for 3 to 5 minutes per side, or until lightly golden brown (it will not be cooked through). Remove the chicken and set aside.

In the same skillet, add the onion and sauté for 3 to 5 minutes, or until softened. Add the garlic, coriander, cinnamon, cumin, paprika, and ginger and sauté for 1 minute. Add the broth and bring to a boil, stirring frequently to dislodge any bits of food that might have stuck to the bottom of the skillet. Return the chicken to the pan, reduce the heat, cover, and simmer for 40 minutes. Add the prunes, carrots, chickpeas, and raisins and stir to combine. Cover and cook for 20 minutes, or until the carrots are tender. Using a slotted spoon, transfer the solids to a serving bowl. Boil the remaining liquid for 1 to 2 minutes to thicken and pour over the chicken, stirring to combine. Top with the almonds and parsley, if desired.

PER SERVING	
Calories	530
Fat	22 g
Saturated fat	4 g
Cholesterol	160 mg
Sodium	470 mg
Carbohydrate	49 g
Dietary fiber	10 g
Sugars	23 g
Protein	37 g
Calcium	140 mg
Potassium	1110 mg

 TIP Prunes (dried plums) are a great digestive aid and contain iron, potassium, and antioxidants.

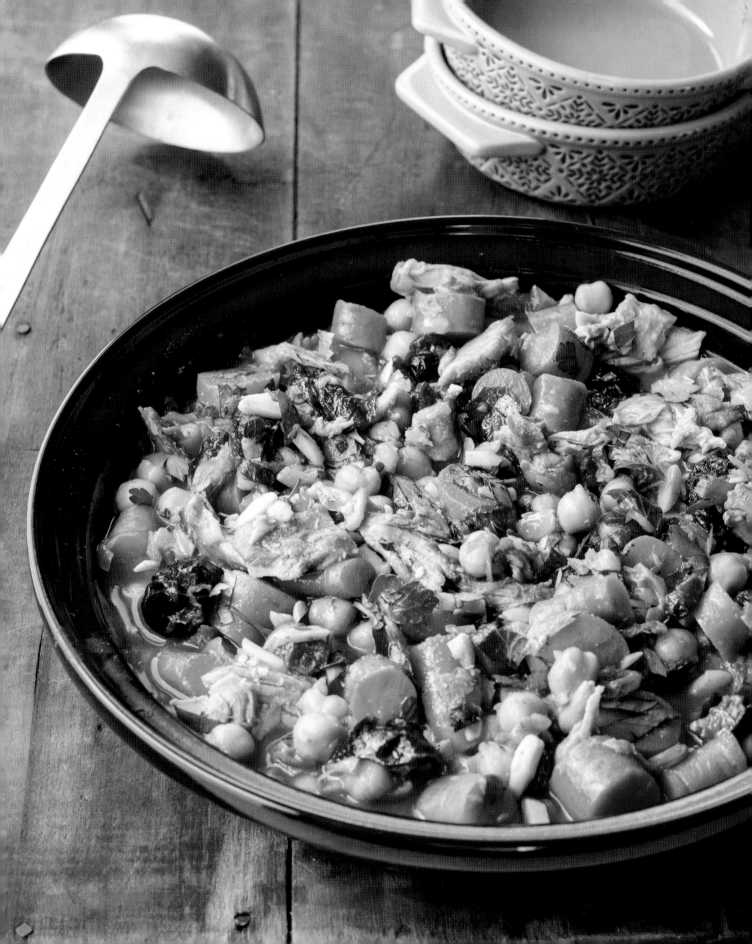

Whole Grain Penne with Roasted Eggplant and Tomatoes

Whole wheat pasta provides two to three times as much fiber as pasta made from refined white flour. The vegetables and chickpeas add more fiber, in addition to providing potassium and vitamins C and A. Cooking the vegetables in the oven instead of on the stovetop makes preparation easy and adds a layer of caramelized, roasted flavor.

Put the water on to boil about twenty minutes before the vegetables are ready, so the sauce and pasta finish at the same time.

4 SERVINGS

1 (1-pound) eggplant, peeled and cut into ½-inch pieces

3 tablespoons olive oil, divided use

Salt and freshly ground black pepper

1 red bell pepper, seeded and cut into ½-inch pieces

1 red onion, cut into 1-inch pieces

4 garlic cloves, quartered

1 (28-ounce) can diced or whole tomatoes, broken up if whole

1 cup canned chickpeas, rinsed and drained

8 ounces whole grain penne

¼ cup thinly sliced fresh basil leaves

¼ cup freshly grated Parmesan cheese

Preheat the oven to 450 degrees.

Place the eggplant in a 9-by-13-inch or larger baking pan. Drizzle with 1 tablespoon of the oil, sprinkle with salt and pepper, and stir to combine. Evenly distribute the eggplant in the pan and bake for 10 minutes. Add the bell pepper, onion, and garlic and stir to combine. Drizzle with 1 tablespoon of the oil and bake for 15 minutes. Add the tomatoes and their juice and the chickpeas and stir to combine. Bake for 20 minutes, stirring after 10 minutes.

Meanwhile, prepare the penne according to the package directions for al dente (just firm).

Reserve ¼ cup of the pasta water before draining. Set aside.

When the vegetables are tender, add the pasta, the remaining 1 tablespoon of oil, and the basil to the baking pan and stir to combine. Season with salt and pepper. If too dry, add reserved pasta water 1 tablespoon at a time, stirring to combine. Top with Parmesan.

PER SERVING	
Calories	480
Fat	14 g
Saturated fat	2.5 g
Cholesterol	5 mg
Sodium	430 mg
Carbohydrate	78 g
Dietary fiber	15 g
Sugars	15 g
Protein	15 g
Calcium	180 mg
Potassium	880 mg

Vegetable, Lentil, and Farro St-oup

This vegetable-lentil medley falls somewhere between a stew and a soup—so voilà, a new word to add to your vocabulary: a "st-oup"!

You can add broth if you prefer a lighter, soup-like dish. For a more fiber-filled stew, add lentils or farro, and adjust the amount of broth to your liking.

6 SERVINGS

2 tablespoons olive oil

1 onion, chopped

1 carrot, sliced

1 celery stalk, sliced

1 small (8-ounce) eggplant, cut into 1/2-inch pieces

2 garlic cloves, minced

1/2 cup dried brown lentils

1/3 cup farro

1 bay leaf

1/4 teaspoon ground cinnamon

4 to 6 cups homemade chicken or vegetable broth (pages 40 or 74) or store-bought reduced-sodium broth

1 (14.5-ounce) can diced tomatoes

Salt and freshly ground black pepper

1 to 2 tablespoons fresh lemon juice, optional

In a large stockpot over medium heat, add the oil. Sauté the onion, carrot, celery, and eggplant for 8 to 10 minutes, or until softened. Add the garlic, lentils, farro, bay leaf, and cinnamon and sauté for 1 minute.

Add 4 cups of broth and tomatoes and their juice and bring to a boil, stirring to combine. Reduce the heat, cover, and simmer for 35 to 45 minutes, or until the lentils and farro are tender, stirring occasionally. If soup is too thick, add broth a half-cup at a time until you achieve the desired consistency. Discard the bay leaf. Season with salt and pepper and lemon juice, if desired.

PER SERVING

Calories	180
Fat	5 g
Saturated fat	0.5 g
Cholesterol	0 mg
Sodium	500 mg
Carbohydrate	26 g
Dietary fiber	8 g
Sugars	6 g
Protein	9 g
Calcium	70 mg
Potassium	640 mg

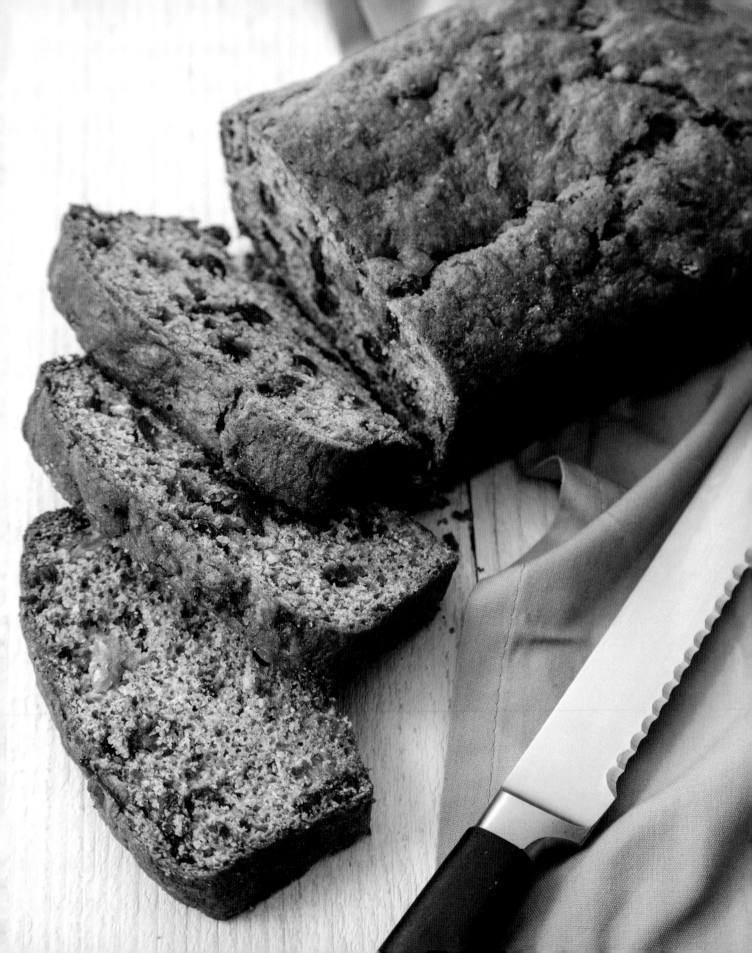

Date and Fruit Bread

Dried dates have experienced a resurgence as a versatile ingredient to add sweetness without refined sugar. This date and fruit bread offers much more fiber than most quick breads, with much of its sweetness coming from natural fruits. The flavor of the bread improves with time, so don't hesitate to bake this a day ahead if time allows.

To easily chop whole dates, lightly coat your knife or kitchen shears with oil or frequently dip in water to prevent the fruit from sticking to the metal. If you are chopping the dates in a food processor, add a few tablespoons of the flour from the recipe to stop them from sticking.

10 TO 12 SLICES

1 cup (4 to 5 ounces) coarsely chopped pitted dates

2/3 cup light brown sugar, firmly packed

1/4 cup (1/2 stick) butter, cut into pieces

3/4 cup boiling water

1 cup all-purpose flour

1 cup whole wheat flour

2 teaspoons baking powder

1 teaspoon baking soda

1/2 teaspoon salt

1 cup assorted dried fruit, such as chopped apricots, raisins, currants, or dried cranberries

2 eggs, beaten

Preheat the oven to 350 degrees. Coat a 9-by-5-by-3-inch loaf pan with nonstick cooking spray. Line the bottom of the pan with parchment paper.

In a large bowl, combine the dates, brown sugar, and butter. Pour the boiling water over the mixture and stir to combine. Set aside for 10 minutes.

Meanwhile, in a bowl, combine both flours, baking powder, baking soda, salt, and dried fruit.

When the butter has melted and the date mixture has cooled, add the eggs and stir to combine. Add the dry ingredients to the date mixture and stir until just combined, scraping down the sides to blend. Do not overmix. Scrape the batter into the pan and smooth the top with a spatula.

Bake for 45 to 55 minutes, or until the top is firm and a toothpick inserted in the center comes out clean. Cool in the pan on a rack for 10 to 15 minutes. Use a knife or spatula to loosen the sides of the loaf from the pan and remove. Cool completely on the rack before slicing.

PER SERVING	
Calories	280
Fat	6 g
Saturated fat	3 g
Cholesterol	50 mg
Sodium	370 mg
Carbohydrate	55 g
Dietary fiber	4 g
Sugars	33 g
Protein	5 g
Calcium	110 mg
Potassium	300 mg

Spinach and Brown Rice "Pie"

This tasty casserole has the flavors of the Greek dish spanakopita, but with less fat and less work. It can be served as a vegetarian entrée or as a side dish with a simple protein. Its Mediterranean flavors are a perfect match for grilled chicken or fish.

This recipe is a great way to use up leftover rice, but if you don't have any on hand, use precooked packaged or quick-cooking rice to save time.

8 TO 10 SERVINGS

2 eggs

2 (10-ounce) packages frozen chopped spinach, thawed, squeezed of excess liquid, and patted dry

3 scallions, thinly sliced

2 cups cooked brown rice or 1 (8.8-ounce) package precooked brown rice

1/2 cup crumbled feta cheese

1/2 cup grated Parmesan cheese

Salt and freshly ground black pepper

3 tablespoons butter

3 tablespoons all-purpose flour

1 2/3 cups milk

Preheat the oven to 350 degrees. Coat a pie plate with nonstick cooking spray.

In a large bowl, beat the eggs. Add the spinach, scallions, rice, feta, and Parmesan cheese and stir well to combine. Sprinkle with salt and pepper.

In a saucepan over low heat, melt the butter. Add the flour and cook until fully incorporated, stirring constantly. Gradually add the milk and bring to a light simmer for 3 to 5 minutes, or until thickened, stirring constantly. Pour the milk mixture over the spinach and stir well to combine. Transfer to the pie plate.

Bake for 25 to 30 minutes or until golden. Let cool for 5 minutes before serving.

PER SERVING

Calories	200
Fat	9 g
Saturated fat	4 g
Cholesterol	75 mg
Sodium	260 mg
Carbohydrate	20 g
Dietary fiber	3 g
Sugars	4 g
Protein	11 g
Calcium	300 mg
Potassium	310 mg

Bulgur Salad with Dried Fruit

Bulgur, also known as cracked wheat, is one of the most fiber-rich grains. Another plus: unlike other grains, it doesn't require a long cooking time. It only needs to be rehydrated in boiling water for about a half-hour.

Get all the other ingredients ready while the bulgur soaks. If you have some fresh Italian parsley on hand, chop one-quarter cup of it and sprinkle over the salad before serving.

If you don't have the time or inclination to squeeze an orange, you can use a high-quality 100 percent orange juice that is freshly squeezed (not from concentrate). Be sure to buy juice that is pasteurized.

6 SERVINGS

1 cup bulgur

1 cup boiling water

1/2 unpeeled apple, chopped

1/4 cup dried sweetened cranberries

1/4 cup golden or brown raisins

2 scallions, thinly sliced

2 tablespoons chopped fresh mint leaves

2 tablespoons olive oil

2 tablespoons fresh lemon juice

2 tablespoons freshly squeezed or 100 percent orange juice

Salt and freshly ground black pepper

2 tablespoons slivered almonds, toasted, optional

In a heatproof bowl, combine the bulgur and water and let stand for 30 minutes. If the mixture is absorbing the water too quickly, add 1 tablespoon or more water.

When the bulgur is tender, add the apple, cranberries, raisins, scallions, and mint. In a bowl, combine the oil, lemon juice, and orange juice. Add to the salad and stir gently to incorporate. Season with salt and pepper. Cover and refrigerate for at least 1 hour. Add the almonds just before serving, if desired.

PER SERVING	
Calories	140
Fat	5 g
Saturated fat	0.5 g
Cholesterol	0 mg
Sodium	5 mg
Carbohydrate	24 g
Dietary fiber	4 g
Sugars	9 g
Protein	3 g
Calcium	20 mg
Potassium	140 mg

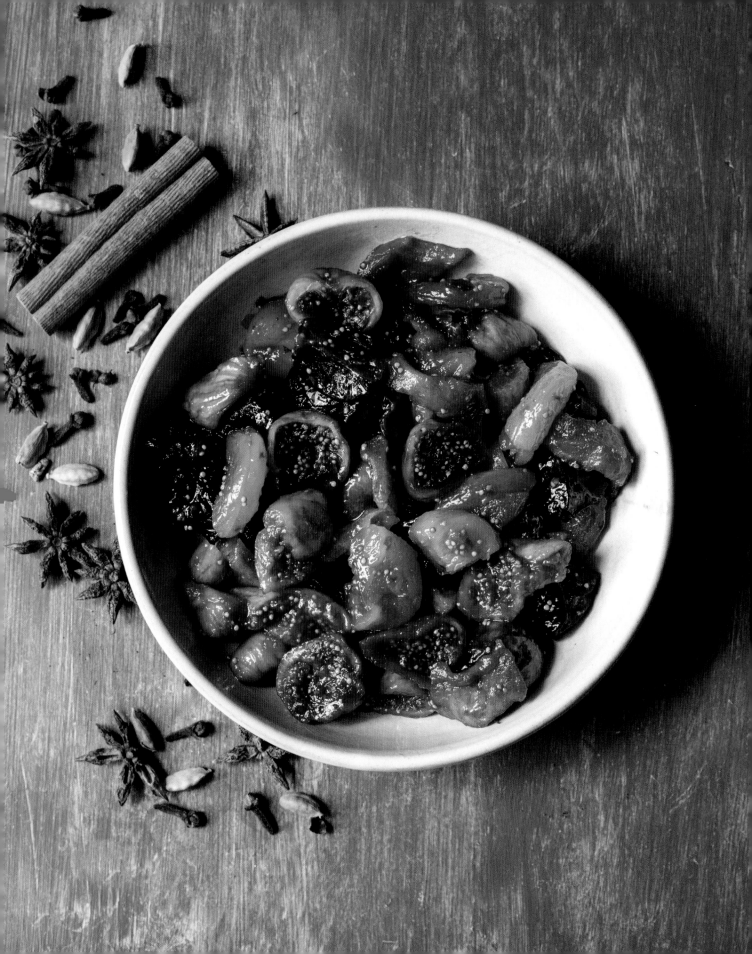

Fig, Apple, and Apricot Compote

This compote, a combination of cooked dried fruit infused with aromatic spices, can be served on its own as a breakfast or dessert, or used as a topping for yogurt or oatmeal. It provides sweetness and toothsome texture with no added processed sugar.

For a softer consistency, add more apple cider and simmer longer to break down the fruit further. If you plan to use the compote primarily as a breakfast topping or spread for crackers or toast, cut the fruit into smaller, bite-sized pieces.

If you have cheesecloth, make a sachet to hold the spices. If not, remove the cloves before adding the fruit, since they can be hard to locate afterward.

If you don't have star anise or cardamom pods on hand, just omit those seasonings.

6 SERVINGS

1 cup pasteurized apple cider or 100 percent apple juice

4 cardamom pods

2 cloves

1 star anise

1 cinnamon stick

1/2 cup dried apple slices

1/2 cup dried apricots, quartered

1/2 cup dried pitted prunes, quartered

1/2 cup dried figs, quartered

1/4 cup dried unsweetened cherries

In a saucepan, combine the apple cider, cardamom pods, cloves, star anise, and cinnamon stick and bring to a boil. Reduce the heat, remove the cloves, add the apples, apricots, prunes, figs, and cherries, and simmer for 8 to 10 minutes, or until the liquid is absorbed, stirring occasionally. Let cool and discard cardamom pods, star anise, and cinnamon stick before serving.

PER SERVING	
Calories	150
Fat	0 g
Saturated fat	0 g
Cholesterol	0 mg
Sodium	10 mg
Carbohydrate	38 g
Dietary fiber	4 g
Sugars	28 g
Protein	1 g
Calcium	40 mg
Potassium	430 mg

 TIP Prunes, apricots, and cherries contain health-promoting phytonutrients.

Date Jam

When puréed, naturally sweet dates make a delicious jam-like paste, ideal to spread on toast or to stir into oatmeal or yogurt when you want to add flavor and fiber without refined sugars.

There are two types of dried dates readily available, Deglet Noor and Medjool. Deglet Noor are thinner with a thicker skin and are commonly sold prepitted in the supermarket. Medjool dates, frequently found in the refrigerated section, are plumper and softer and have a creamy texture. They are also much more expensive. Deglet Noor dates work well here because they are softened in boiling water before being puréed.

If you want an even softer, more mixable jam, increase the amount of water. For stronger flavor, add a pinch or two of cinnamon.

Store the jam in a lidded container in the refrigerator.

12 SERVINGS ———————————————————————

1 cup pitted Deglet Noor dates   ½ to 1 cup boiling water

In a bowl, combine the dates and ½ cup of the boiling water, pushing the dates down to submerge them in the water. Set aside for 5 to 10 minutes. Transfer the mixture to a food processor and purée until smooth, scraping down the blade and sides to blend, and adding water, 1 tablespoon at a time, until it reaches the desired consistency.

PER SERVING

Calories	35
Fat	0 g
Saturated fat	0 g
Cholesterol	0 mg
Sodium	0 mg
Carbohydrate	9 g
Dietary fiber	1 g
Sugars	8 g
Protein	0 g
Calcium	10 mg
Potassium	80 mg

Multigrain Almond Butter and Date Jam Sandwich

Date purée offers the sweetness of a jam without any processed sugar, while the almond butter provides protein and stands up to a dense multigrain roll. If you can't find a roll, substitute two slices of lightly toasted multigrain bread.

1 SERVING

2 tablespoons Date Jam (page 114)

Pinch or 2 ground cinnamon

2 tablespoons almond butter

1 (3- to 4-inch) whole wheat multigrain roll, split in half

In a bowl, combine the date jam and cinnamon. Set aside.

Spread the almond butter on the bottom of the roll. Top with the date jam and remaining piece of roll.

PER SERVING

Calories	330
Fat	20 g
Saturated fat	1.5 g
Cholesterol	0 mg
Sodium	200 mg
Carbohydrate	34 g
Dietary fiber	7 g
Sugars	12 g
Protein	10 g
Calcium	160 mg
Potassium	420 mg

Crunchy Roasted Lemon-Garlic Chickpeas

This protein-filled snack is great when you feel like something crunchy to munch on. If your sense of taste is dulled, use extra garlic powder, onion powder, or salt; for even more intense seasoning, sprinkle with smoked paprika or curry powder.

Line the baking sheet with parchment paper for easy cleanup.

4 SERVINGS

1 (15-ounce) can chickpeas, rinsed, drained, and patted dry

2 teaspoons olive oil

Zest of 1 lemon

Scant ¼ teaspoon garlic powder

Scant ¼ teaspoon onion powder

Kosher or sea salt

Preheat the oven to 400 degrees.

Spread the chickpeas in a single layer on a rimmed baking sheet. Bake for 30 to 40 minutes, or until the chickpeas are golden brown and crunchy, shaking the baking sheet occasionally during cooking to redistribute the chickpeas.

Meanwhile, in a bowl large enough to hold the chickpeas, combine the oil, lemon zest, garlic powder, and onion powder.

Toss the hot chickpeas with the oil mixture and sprinkle with salt.

PER SERVING	
Calories	120
Fat	4 g
Saturated fat	0.5 g
Cholesterol	0 mg
Sodium	110 mg
Carbohydrate	17 g
Dietary fiber	5 g
Sugars	3 g
Protein	6 g
Calcium	30 mg
Potassium	190 mg

 TIP Chickpeas are also known as garbanzo beans.

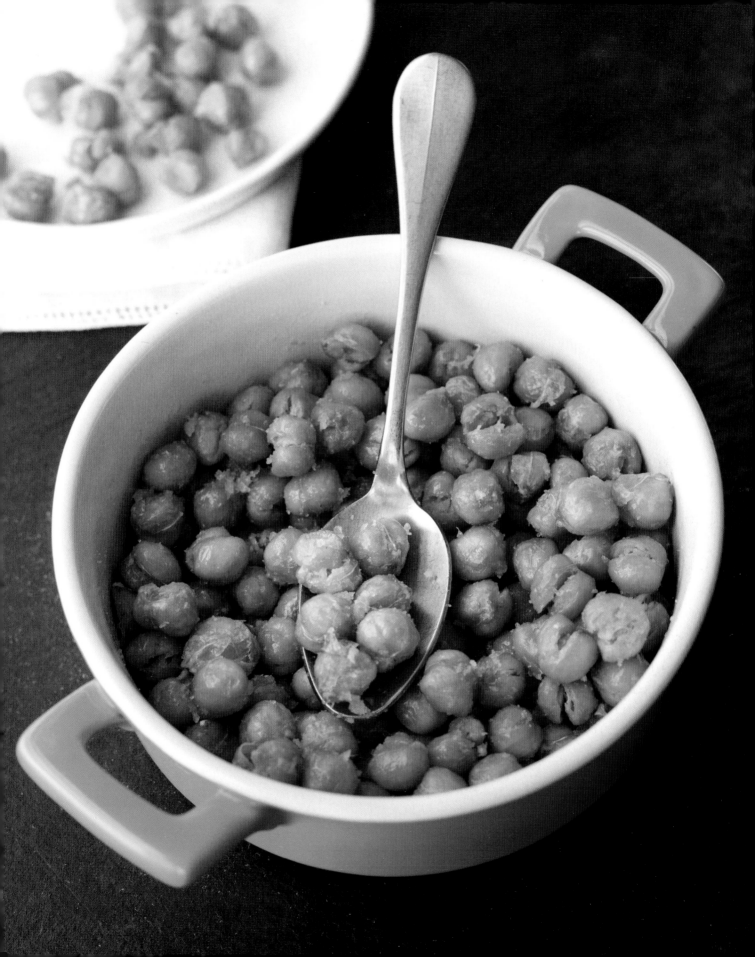

Fiber-Filled Trail Mix

Trail mixes can provide calories when you need to eat but are not up to eating a traditional meal. This mix is an easy and filling snack that also provides fiber and protein through a combination of dried fruits, seeds, and nuts.

11 SERVINGS

2 cups air-popped popcorn

1 cup high-fiber cereal, such as Mini Wheats or Wheat Chex

1/2 cup roasted salted peanuts or almonds

1/2 cup dried apricots

1/2 cup dried cherries or raisins

1/2 cup dried sweetened cranberries

1/2 cup roasted sunflower seeds, shelled

In a container with an airtight lid, combine the popcorn, cereal, peanuts, apricots, cherries, cranberries, and sunflower seeds.

PER SERVING	
Calories	150
Fat	6 g
Saturated fat	1 g
Cholesterol	0 mg
Sodium	55 mg
Carbohydrate	23 g
Dietary fiber	3 g
Sugars	14 g
Protein	4 g
Calcium	20 mg
Potassium	220 mg

 TIP This is a good snack to keep in your car or take to treatment.

Honey-Bran Muffins

These fiber-filled muffins, sweetened with honey and molasses, are good to have on hand for breakfast or when you need a snack on the run.

For added protein and fiber, split a muffin in half, toast, and top with peanut or almond butter and/or Date Jam (page 114).

Wheat bran can be found in the baking or health section of most supermarkets.

12 MUFFINS

1 1/2 cups wheat bran

3/4 cups all-purpose flour

3/4 cups whole wheat flour

1/4 cup light brown sugar, firmly packed

2 teaspoons baking powder

1/2 teaspoon baking soda

1/2 teaspoon salt

1 cup raisins

2 eggs

1 cup buttermilk

1/4 cup (1/2 stick) butter, melted and slightly cooled

1/4 cup honey

1/4 cup molasses

Preheat the oven to 400 degrees. Coat a muffin tin with nonstick cooking spray or fill with liners.

In a bowl, combine the bran, both flours, brown sugar, baking powder, baking soda, salt, and raisins. Make a well in the center. Set aside.

In a bowl, beat the eggs. Add the buttermilk, butter, honey, and molasses and mix until blended. Pour into the dry ingredients' well. Stir until just combined, scraping down the sides to blend. Do not overmix. Spoon the batter into prepared muffin cups, dividing evenly.

Bake for 18 to 20 minutes, or until tops are firm. Cool in the tin on a rack for 15 minutes before removing the muffins to the rack to cool completely.

PER SERVING
(ONE MUFFIN)

Calories	220
Fat	5 g
Saturated fat	3 g
Cholesterol	40 mg
Sodium	280 mg
Carbohydrate	42 g
Dietary fiber	5 g
Sugars	24 g
Protein	5 g
Calcium	120 mg
Potassium	370 mg

 TIP Spray a measuring cup with nonstick spray before filling it with sticky substances such as honey or molasses to make the liquid slip right out.

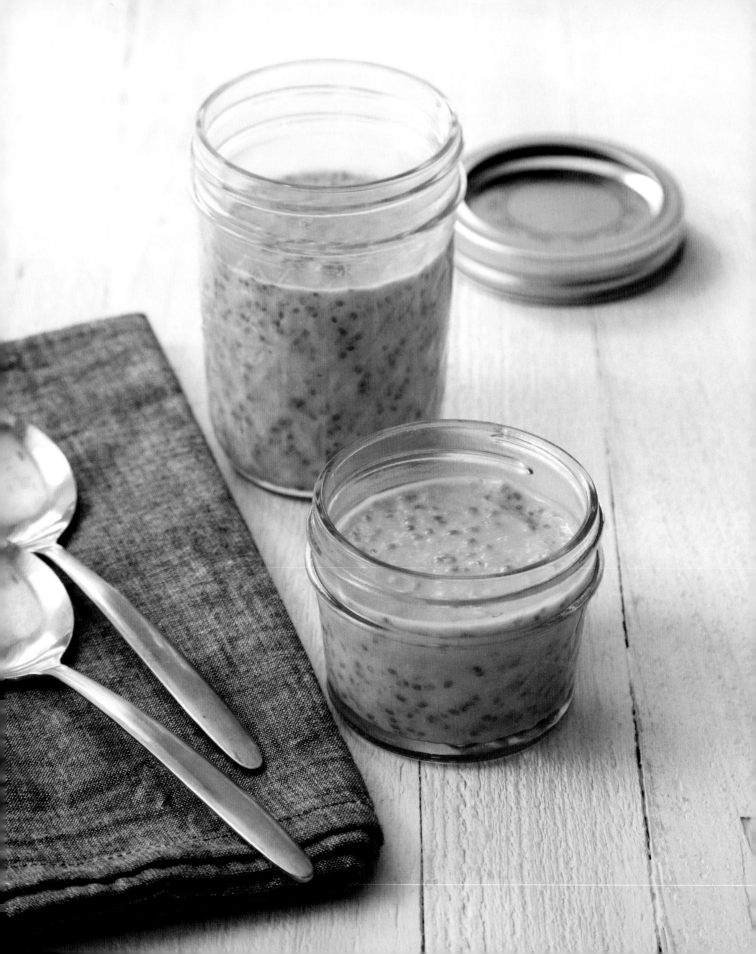

Raspberry Chia Pudding

Chia pudding is a food craze that doesn't seem to be slowing. Tiny chia seeds, often found in the health food section of your supermarket, are rich in fiber, protein, calcium, and magnesium. Soaking the seeds in liquid softens them so that they function as a thickener. When added to puréed fruit and coconut milk, the result is a light, creamy, and refreshing pudding, much like tapioca in texture.

Chia puddings should sit for at least four hours or overnight to allow the seeds time to absorb as much liquid as possible to ensure they are soft enough that they don't irritate your throat. This is especially important if you are having trouble swallowing or have any throat sensitivity.

For an even creamier texture, mix the finished pudding with yogurt or layer it with plain or vanilla yogurt for a parfait. If you want to add calories, use full-fat coconut milk. If weight gain is an issue, choose the light variety.

If desired, garnish the pudding with additional fresh raspberries before eating.

4 SERVINGS

½ cup unsweetened coconut milk, well shaken

½ cup fresh or frozen raspberries, defrosted

2 to 3 tablespoons maple syrup, agave nectar, or honey

2 tablespoons chia seeds

In a blender, combine the coconut milk, raspberries, and 2 tablespoons of the maple syrup until smooth. Taste and add more maple syrup, if desired. Pour into a bowl and add the chia seeds, stirring well to combine. Leave in the bowl or transfer to individual ramekins for serving. Cover with plastic wrap and refrigerate for at least 4 hours or overnight.

PER SERVING	
Calories	60
Fat	2.5 g
Saturated fat	1 g
Cholesterol	0 mg
Sodium	0 mg
Carbohydrate	8 g
Dietary fiber	3 g
Sugars	4 g
Protein	1 g
Calcium	60 mg
Potassium	70 mg

 TIP You can substitute unsweetened (plain) almond milk for coconut milk.

Granola with Almond, Apples, and Ginger

There is a misconception that anything labeled "granola" is a health food. Unfortunately, even though heart-healthy oats are usually the main ingredient, most commercial granolas are loaded with added sugars and oil. This homemade version uses applesauce, dried fruit, and a small amount of honey to add a hint of sweetness. The coating darkens as it bakes, so watch to make sure the granola isn't overbrowning, especially if your oven has a tendency to run hot.

You can add any dried fruit you prefer (or none!) during the last ten to fifteen minutes of cooking; just be sure to stir the mixture every five minutes for even baking.

Flaxseeds contain fiber and omega-3 essential fatty acids. To get more of the nutrients, it is recommended to grind them first (a coffee grinder works great) to prevent them from passing through the intestinal tract undigested.

Don't be concerned if the granola is a little soft after baking. It will continue to crisp up as it cools.

12 TO 14 SERVINGS

½ cup unsweetened applesauce

⅓ cup honey

2 tablespoons canola oil

1 teaspoon vanilla extract

1 teaspoon ground cinnamon

1 teaspoon ground ginger

3 cups old-fashioned rolled oats

½ cup slivered, sliced, or chopped almonds

2 tablespoons ground flaxseeds

½ cup raisins or dried cherries

¼ cup chopped crystallized ginger

½ cup chopped dried apples

Preheat the oven to 325 degrees. Line a rimmed baking sheet with parchment paper or aluminum foil.

In a bowl, combine the applesauce, honey, oil, vanilla, cinnamon, and ginger. Add the oats, almonds, and flaxseeds and stir to combine. Spread the mixture evenly on the baking sheet. Bake for 30 to 35 minutes, stirring once. Remove from the oven and stir to redistribute the mixture. Bake for 15 minutes.

Reduce the heat to 300 degrees. Remove the tray from the oven, add the raisins and crystallized ginger, and stir to combine. Bake for 5 minutes. Add the dried apples and stir to combine. Bake for 5 to 10 minutes, or until golden brown, stirring every 5 minutes to prevent burning. Cool completely before storing.

PER SERVING	
Calories	210
Fat	7 g
Saturated fat	0.5 g
Cholesterol	0 mg
Sodium	5 mg
Carbohydrate	35 g
Dietary fiber	4 g
Sugars	18 g
Protein	4 g
Calcium	30 mg
Potassium	200 mg

Tuna Salad

This colorful mayonnaise-based salad, served on a bed of greens, is full of healthful vegetables.

Add whichever embellishments you enjoy: olives, artichoke hearts, hard-boiled eggs, and cucumber are good options.

3 SERVINGS

1 (5-ounce) can white tuna packed in water, drained

2 teaspoons regular or reduced-fat mayonnaise

1/2 teaspoon Dijon mustard

1 tablespoon red onion, finely chopped

1/2 red, green, or yellow bell pepper, seeded and finely chopped

1/2 celery stalk, finely chopped

1/4 cup matchstick carrots, finely chopped

Salt and freshly ground black pepper

6 cups mixed salad greens

2 tomatoes, cut into quarters (or eighths if large)

In a bowl, flake the tuna. Add the mayonnaise and mustard and stir to combine. Add the onion, bell pepper, celery, and carrots and stir gently to incorporate. Season with salt and pepper.

Divide the greens and tomatoes on three plates and top with a scoop of the tuna mixture.

PER SERVING

Calories	120
Fat	4 g
Saturated fat	1 g
Cholesterol	20 mg
Sodium	220 mg
Carbohydrate	9 g
Dietary fiber	3 g
Sugars	6 g
Protein	12 g
Calcium	60 mg
Potassium	650 mg

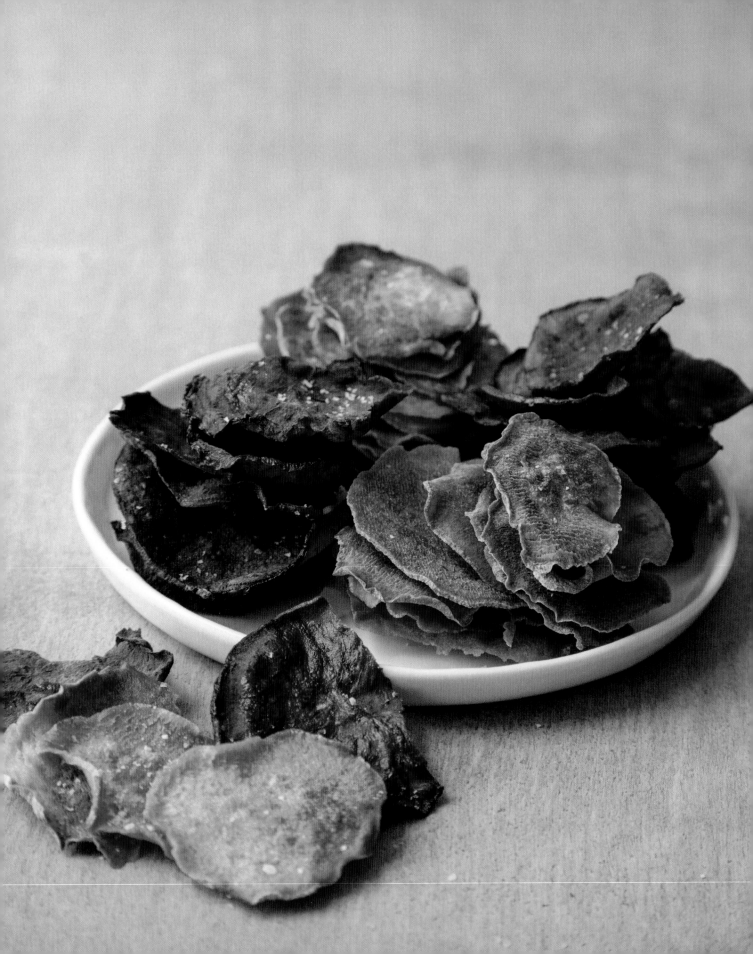

Baked Sweet Potato and Beet Chips

When you want a snack and don't want to feel deprived, why not try healthier chips made from fiber-filled, nutrient-rich sweet potatoes and/or beets. They provide the crunch and saltiness of traditional chips but are better for you.

Because the vegetables need to be sliced very thinly for even baking, using a mandoline (a type of handheld slicer) or a very sharp knife is recommended. Oddly, even when uniformly sliced, the chips still cook at slightly different rates. Watch carefully and remove them, especially the sweet potato chips, when they are done, leaving the others to continue cooking. Don't worry about spacing too much when placing the slices on the baking tray. The chips will shrink dramatically during cooking.

Lining your baking sheets with aluminum foil speeds cleanup and prevents sticking. Use a basting brush to lightly spread the oil on the baking sheet and the chips.

Sweet Potato Chips

2 TO 3 SERVINGS

2 teaspoons olive oil

1 sweet potato, peeled and sliced ⅛-inch thick

Kosher or sea salt

Preheat the oven to 350 degrees. Brush two rimmed baking sheets lightly with oil. Arrange the potato slices in a single layer on the baking sheets, brush with the remaining oil, and sprinkle lightly with salt.

Bake for 20 minutes. Remove from the oven, flip the chips, and sprinkle lightly with salt. Bake for 30 to 40 minutes, or until darkened and crispy, checking every 5 minutes during the last 15 minutes of cooking, and transferring chips that are done to a plate.

PER SERVING	
Calories	90
Fat	5 g
Saturated fat	1 g
Cholesterol	0 mg
Sodium	20 mg
Carbohydrate	11 g
Dietary fiber	2 g
Sugars	3 g
Protein	1 g
Calcium	20 mg
Potassium	250 mg

Recipe continued

Beet Chips

2 TO 3 SERVINGS

2 teaspoons olive oil

2 beets, peeled and sliced 1/8-inch thick

Kosher or sea salt

Preheat the oven to 350 degrees. Brush two rimmed baking sheets lightly with oil. Arrange the beet slices in a single layer on the baking sheets, brush with the remaining oil, and sprinkle lightly with salt.

Bake for 30 minutes. Reduce the heat to 225 degrees. Remove from the oven, flip the chips, and sprinkle lightly with salt. Bake for 60 minutes, or until crispy, checking every 5 minutes during the last 15 minutes of cooking, and transferring chips that are done to a plate.

PER SERVING

Calories	70
Fat	5 g
Saturated fat	1 g
Cholesterol	0 mg
Sodium	55 mg
Carbohydrate	7 g
Dietary fiber	1 g
Sugars	6 g
Protein	1 g
Calcium	10 mg
Potassium	220 mg

NOTES

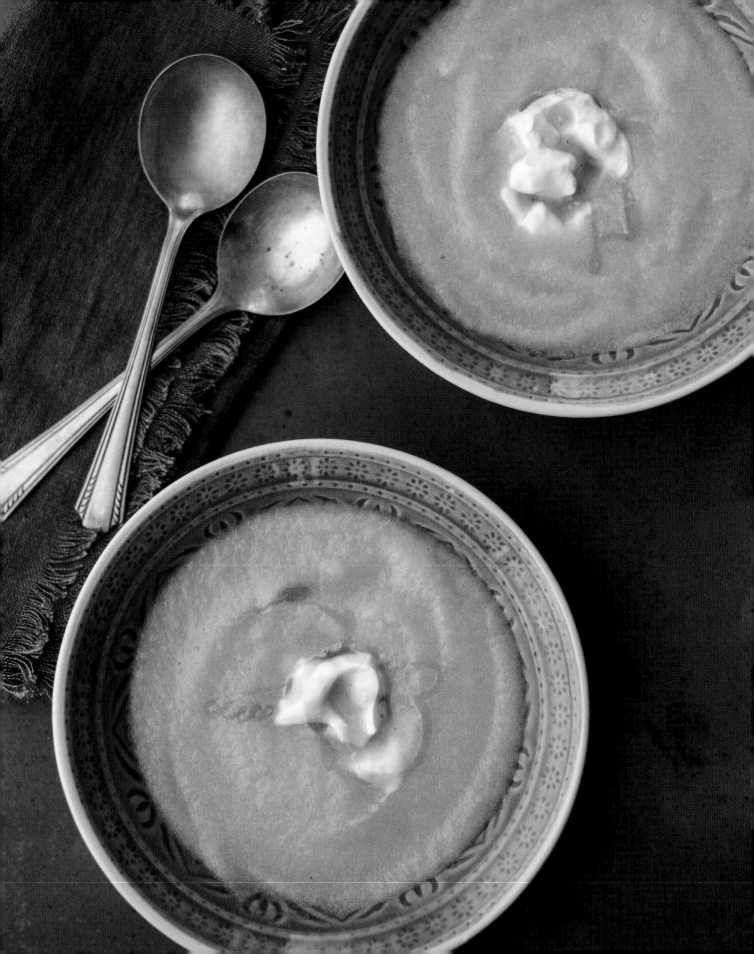

TS TROUBLE SWALLOWING

Creamy Avocado Soup

Fresh Mint Milk Shake

Pressure Cooker Potato-Leek Soup

Egg Drop Soup

Chilled Cucumber and Yogurt Soup

Golden Milk

Chai Applesauce

Cranberry-Pear Compote

Roasted Cauliflower Soup

Cantaloupe-Peach Soup

Sweet Potato and Cashew Purée

Mango Lassi

Cranberry-Lime Granita

Vanilla Juice Glass Pudding

PB and Banana Smoothie

Chilled Beet Soup with Yogurt-Dill Swirl

Roasted Root Vegetable Soup

White Bean and Roasted Garlic Dip

Love Your Greens Shake

DIFFICULTY SWALLOWING (DYSPHAGIA) OR PAIN WHEN SWALLOWING CAN BE CAUSED BY DIFFERENT TYPES OF CANCER OR CANCER TREATMENT. Sometimes the cancer itself may block or obstruct the esophagus, making it difficult for food or liquids to pass. Swallowing is critical to getting adequate nutrition. These are symptoms that suggest you may be experiencing dysphagia:

- Inability to drink liquids without coughing or choking, also known as aspiration

- Difficulty or pain with swallowing hard, coarse, or rough foods

- Feeling like solid foods get stuck or lodged in your throat and will not pass

Some people may be referred to a swallowing specialist such as a speech-language pathologist (SLP) for individualized help and therapy. Doing swallowing exercises and adjusting the consistency and texture of the foods and liquids you consume may be helpful and make it safer for you to swallow.

If you have dysphagia, bland, moist soft or semisoft foods will most likely be easier to chew and swallow. Your doctor may also refer you to a registered dietitian for safe food options and ways to thicken or soften food. These suggestions may help:

- Eat small, more frequent meals and snacks.

- Avoid rough-textured foods such as dry toast, crackers, pretzels, granola, raw vegetables and fruits, or fried or baked foods with rough exteriors or coatings.

- Eat soft protein-rich foods such as casseroles, cream soups, soft cooked beans or peas, soft scrambled eggs, ground or puréed meats and poultry, poached or baked fish, cottage cheese, yogurt without pieces of fruit, custards, puddings, ice cream, smoothies, and milk shakes.

- Other soft foods include mashed potatoes, cooked cereals, cold cereals softened in milk, pancakes and waffles, pasta, soft cooked vegetables, well-cooked vegetable soups, applesauce, bananas, avocado, cooked fruit, juices and nectars, and gelatin.

- Blend, purée, or liquefy foods in a blender to make them easier to eat. Add enough liquid (broth, juice, or milk) to achieve the desired consistency.

For some people, thicker liquids are more easily tolerated than thin liquids. There are several ways to thicken liquids and soften foods:

■ Add tapioca, flour, or cornstarch to cool water. Then mix into the liquid before heating so that the thickener dissolves completely.

■ Use commercial thickeners found at your local drugstore or pharmacy to adjust the thickness of a food or liquid. Follow the label instructions.

■ Use puréed vegetables or instant potatoes in soups.

■ Use baby rice cereal to make liquids thicker.

■ Mix one tablespoon of unflavored gelatin in two cups of liquid until dissolved and then pour over the food. (Consult the package directions to be sure.) Allow the food to sit until saturated.

CONTACT YOUR DOCTOR IN THESE SITUATIONS:

■ You are unable to drink liquids without coughing or choking. This is a more serious concern and should be brought to the attention of your health care team immediately.

■ It feels like food is getting stuck in your throat.

For more information about managing difficulty with swallowing, visit the American Cancer Society website at cancer.org or call 800-227-2345.

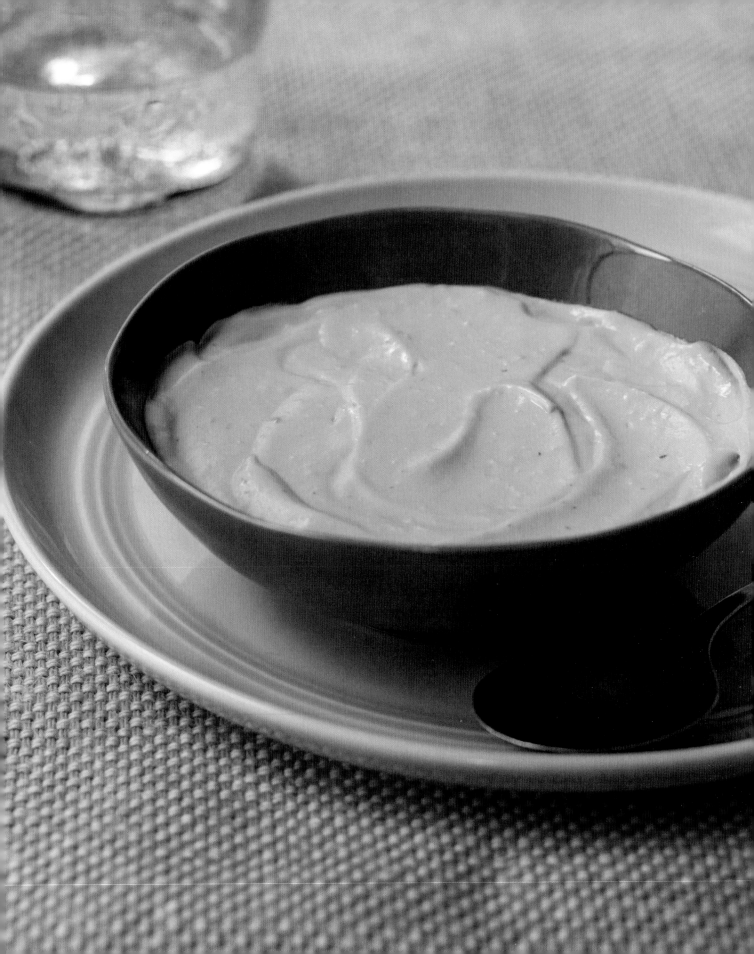

Creamy Avocado Soup

When you're having trouble swallowing or your mouth is sensitive, a creamy, chilled soup can be calming.

For milder garlic flavor, the garlic clove is blanched in boiling water for one minute before combining it with the other ingredients. If you like more assertive garlic flavor, you can add it to the mixture raw.

If you are experiencing mouth sores, omit the lime juice. Or start with one teaspoon and add more, if palatable.

4 SERVINGS

1 garlic clove

3 ripe avocados, halved and pitted

1 1/2 to 2 cups buttermilk

1/2 cup plain Greek yogurt

1 to 2 tablespoons fresh lime juice

1/2 to 1 teaspoon salt

In a small saucepan, bring 2 inches of water to a boil. Add the garlic and cook for 1 minute. Remove and set aside.

In a food processor or blender, scrape in the avocado flesh. Add the blanched garlic, 1 1/2 cups of the buttermilk, yogurt, 1 tablespoon of the lime juice, and 1/2 teaspoon of the salt and process until smooth, scraping down the blade and sides to blend. If the soup is too thick, add buttermilk to the desired consistency. Taste and add salt and lime juice, if desired. Transfer to a bowl and press a piece of plastic wrap on top of the surface of the soup. Refrigerate for at least 2 hours.

PER SERVING	
Calories	250
Fat	19 g
Saturated fat	3.5 g
Cholesterol	7 mg
Sodium	360 mg
Carbohydrate	16 g
Dietary fiber	8 g
Sugars	6 g
Protein	8 g
Calcium	150 mg
Potassium	730 mg

TIP For the family (or when the side effect has resolved), garnish with 2 tablespoons finely chopped fresh mint, dill, or cilantro or sprinkle a few cubes of avocado or chopped cherry tomatoes on top.

Fresh Mint Milk Shake

When you need extra calories and want refreshing, unadulterated flavor, try this yummy shake made with milk simmered and steeped with fresh mint.

If you want stronger mint flavor, add a few drops of peppermint extract during blending.

1 SERVING

3/4 cup milk

3/4 cup fresh mint leaves

1 cup vanilla ice cream

Peppermint extract, optional

In a saucepan over medium heat, combine the milk and mint and bring to a simmer for 1 to 2 minutes. Transfer the mixture to a container and refrigerate for 30 or more minutes.

When ready to serve, strain the milk into a blender, pushing down with a spoon to extract all the liquid. Add the ice cream and blend until smooth. For stronger peppermint flavor, add a shake or two of peppermint extract, if desired.

PER SERVING

Calories	350
Fat	19 g
Saturated fat	11 g
Cholesterol	70 mg
Sodium	160 mg
Carbohydrate	37 g
Dietary fiber	1 g
Sugars	35 g
Protein	9 g
Calcium	320 mg
Potassium	440 mg

Pressure Cooker Potato-Leek Soup

This thick root vegetable soup is a respite for those experiencing swallowing problems or mouth sores. The parsnip gives the soup a thick consistency, which can be easily thinned with broth, water, or—if you desire a creamier texture and more calcium and calories—cream or half-and-half. For added calories, melt shredded Cheddar cheese into the soup after puréeing.

A pressure cooker is used here, but it can also be cooked on the stovetop or in a slow cooker. For stovetop cooking, use the same initial directions, including sautéing the leeks, and simmer, partially covered, for one to two hours, or until vegetables are softened. For a slow cooker, add all the ingredients together and cook on desired setting. This soup uses less broth than many soups, so the liquid will barely cover the vegetables. If using a slow cooker, stir the mixture every two or three hours.

Check your pressure cooker manual for recommended cooking and cooling methods. Every cooker varies slightly.

8 SERVINGS

1 tablespoon olive oil

2 leeks, white and light green parts only, thinly sliced

1 large russet potato, peeled and cut into 1-inch pieces

1 pound parsnips, cut into 1-inch pieces

1 carrot, cut into 1-inch pieces

2 garlic cloves, sliced

1 sprig fresh thyme or 1/2 teaspoon dried thyme

4 cups homemade chicken or vegetable broth (pages 40 or 74) or store-bought reduced-sodium broth

Salt and freshly ground black pepper

In a pressure cooker over medium heat, add the oil. Sauté the leeks for 3 to 5 minutes, or until softened. Add the potato, parsnips, carrot, garlic, and thyme and stir to combine. Add the broth and cook on high pressure for 10 minutes. Run the water around the edges of the lid to release pressure after cooking (also known as cold-water quick release) or release pressure according to your cooker's manufacturers' directions.

Discard the thyme sprig. Purée the soup with an immersion blender, a blender, or food processor. Season with salt and pepper.

PER SERVING	
Calories	110
Fat	2.5 g
Saturated fat	0 g
Cholesterol	5 mg
Sodium	260 mg
Carbohydrate	21 g
Dietary fiber	3 g
Sugars	4 g
Protein	3 g
Calcium	40 mg
Potassium	400 mg

TIP Be very careful when blending soup in a blender or food processor. Let the soup cool slightly, don't fill the container more than two-thirds full, and secure the lid well before blending.

Egg Drop Soup

This soup has "soothing" written all over it. The mild broth gets a creamy consistency from ribbons of gently cooked eggs. The eggs also provide protein, fat, and other important nutrients. Because the broth is one of only a few ingredients, try to use homemade broth (page 40) for the best flavor.

Use a microplane to finely grate the ginger, to make sure it is as smooth as possible for easy swallowing.

4 SERVINGS

4 cups homemade chicken broth (page 40) or store-bought reduced-sodium broth

2 teaspoons reduced-sodium soy sauce or tamari

¼ teaspoon finely grated fresh ginger

1 tablespoon cornstarch

3 eggs, beaten

Salt

Freshly ground black pepper, optional

In a large saucepan over high heat, bring the broth, soy sauce, and ginger to a boil. Reduce the heat to low. Remove ½ cup of warm broth and gradually add to the cornstarch, whisking until smooth and completely combined. Add the mixture back to the pot, stirring constantly to prevent clumping.

Drizzle the egg into the saucepan, stirring constantly. Season with salt and pepper, if desired.

PER SERVING	
Calories	80
Fat	4.5 g
Saturated fat	1.5 g
Cholesterol	145 mg
Sodium	640 mg
Carbohydrate	3 g
Dietary fiber	0 g
Sugars	0 g
Protein	7 g
Calcium	30 mg
Potassium	70 mg

 TIP For the family (or when the side effect has resolved), add thinly sliced scallions, sautéed mushrooms, chopped cooked chicken, or cooked rice for a more substantial soup.

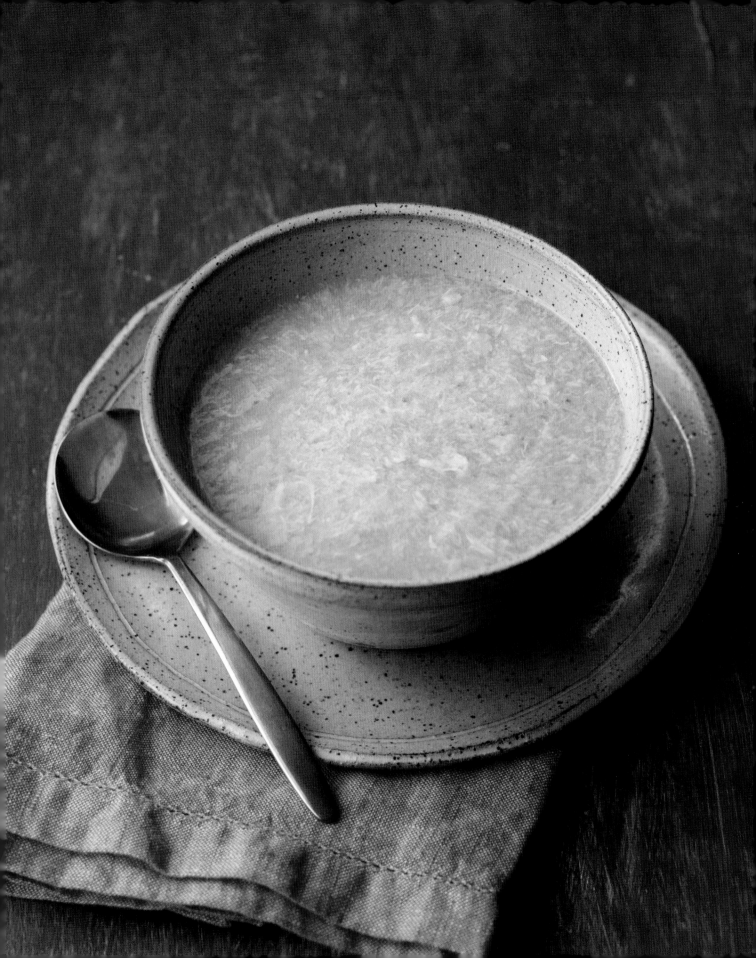

Chilled Cucumber and Yogurt Soup

This cold soup offers subtle flavors in a refreshing way, especially if your mouth is sensitive to heat. To seed the cucumber, simply slice in half lengthwise and use a spoon to scoop out the seeds from the middle. Some tiny bits of cucumber will remain in the final soup.

Use full-fat yogurt if you are trying to gain weight. This soup is also good for weight reduction, if made with nonfat yogurt.

6 SERVINGS

1 large garlic clove

2 tablespoons fresh dill, thick stems removed

3 medium cucumbers, peeled, seeded, and chopped coarsely (about 4 cups)

2 cups plain nonfat yogurt or Greek yogurt

2 cups water

1 tablespoon olive oil

1 tablespoon honey

2 teaspoons salt

1 teaspoon ground black pepper

In a food processor, with the motor running, drop in the garlic and dill and purée. Stop the machine, add the cucumbers, and pulse until finely chopped. Add the yogurt, water, oil, honey, salt, and pepper and pulse 2 or 3 times just to combine. Do not overprocess.

Transfer to a large bowl. Cover and refrigerate for at least 2 hours. If the soup thickens too much, dilute with ice cubes.

PER SERVING	
Calories	80
Fat	2.5 g
Saturated fat	0 g
Cholesterol	5 mg
Sodium	830 mg
Carbohydrate	11 g
Dietary fiber	0.5 g
Sugars	9 g
Protein	5 g
Calcium	180 mg
Potassium	330 mg

 TIP If garlic is bothersome, you can leave it out.

Golden Milk

This smooth and silky drink has gentle flavor and stomach-soothing fresh turmeric and ginger. Look for fresh turmeric in the grocery store near the ginger or, if necessary, substitute one teaspoon ground turmeric.

1 SERVING

1 cup almond milk

1 (1-inch piece) fresh turmeric, peeled and coarsely chopped

1 (1/2-inch) slice fresh ginger, peeled and coarsely chopped

1 to 2 tablespoons honey

Pinch or 2 freshly ground black pepper

Pinch or 2 ground cinnamon

In a blender, combine the almond milk, turmeric, ginger, 1 tablespoon of the honey, pepper, and cinnamon and process until smooth. Transfer to a saucepan and warm over medium heat, stirring frequently. Strain the mixture through a fine mesh sieve into a mug, pushing down with a spoon to extract all the liquid. Taste and add honey, if desired.

PER SERVING

Calories	110
Fat	2.5 g
Saturated fat	0 g
Cholesterol	0 mg
Sodium	180 mg
Carbohydrate	20 g
Dietary fiber	0.5 g
Sugars	17 g
Protein	1 g
Calcium	460 mg
Potassium	250 mg

TIP Some high-speed blenders, such as the Vitamix, have a heat setting in addition to blending settings. This drink can also be heated in a blender of that type.

Chai Applesauce

When you are having trouble swallowing, any applesauce, especially one flavored with warming spices, can be comforting. This version is slightly chunky; if a softer consistency is desired, cook longer and use a potato masher to further break down the applesauce.

For a slightly different flavor profile, substitute one or two ripe pears for apples, if you have them on hand.

4 SERVINGS

4 Granny Smith or Yellow Delicious apples, peeled, cored, and cut into ½-inch pieces

¼ cup light brown sugar

2 tablespoons fresh lemon juice

½ teaspoon ground cinnamon

½ teaspoon ground ginger

¼ teaspoon ground nutmeg

¼ teaspoon ground cardamom

Pinch or 2 cloves

Pinch or 2 salt

In a saucepan over medium heat, combine the apples, brown sugar, and lemon juice and cook until it begins to sizzle or simmer (there's not much liquid, so it might not come to a full simmer). Stir in the cinnamon, ginger, nutmeg, cardamom, cloves, and salt and stir to combine. Reduce the heat to low, cover, and cook for 5 to 10 minutes, or until the apples release their juices and are very tender.

PER SERVING	
Calories	100
Fat	0 g
Saturated fat	0 g
Cholesterol	0 mg
Sodium	45 mg
Carbohydrate	26 g
Dietary fiber	2 g
Sugars	22 g
Protein	0 g
Calcium	20 mg
Potassium	140 mg

 TIP If you have a sore mouth or throat, omit the spices and lemon juice.

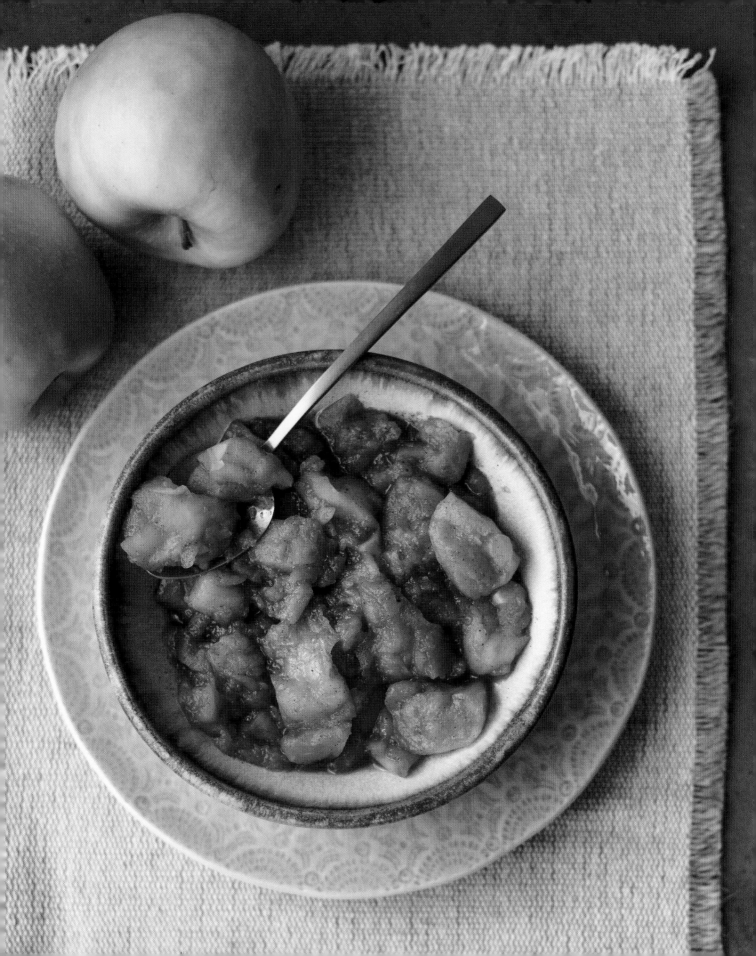

Cranberry-Pear Compote

In cooler months when you want to jazz up your breakfast with fruit but fresh berries are not in season, make a compote from autumnal favorites cranberries and pears. This mixture is equally good on its own or as a topping for yogurt, cottage cheese, or oatmeal.

After cooking, the mixture sets up to a pudding-like consistency, making it a good choice when you are looking for flavorful soft foods. If the mixture is too thick, add juice or mix with plain or vanilla yogurt until it's the right consistency for easy swallowing. For a smoother texture, run it through a food processor.

If you have mouth sores or a sore throat, substitute apple juice for the orange juice, which might be too acidic.

If using frozen cranberries, there's no need to defrost them before cooking.

5 SERVINGS

2 cups fresh or frozen cranberries

1 pear, peeled, cored, and chopped

½ cup freshly squeezed or 100 percent orange juice

1 to 2 tablespoons light brown sugar

In a saucepan over medium-high heat, bring the cranberries, pear, and orange juice to a boil. Reduce the heat, add 1 tablespoon of the brown sugar, and simmer for 5 to 8 minutes, or until the cranberries soften, stirring occasionally. Taste and add brown sugar, if desired. Let cool until the juices thicken and serve as is or purée for a smoother texture.

PER SERVING

Calories	60
Fat	0 g
Saturated fat	0 g
Cholesterol	0 mg
Sodium	0 mg
Carbohydrate	14 g
Dietary fiber	3 g
Sugars	9 g
Protein	0.5 g
Calcium	10 mg
Potassium	130 mg

Roasted Cauliflower Soup

This creamy, mild soup requires almost no labor. The main flavoring comes simply from the caramelization of the roasted cauliflower. A hint of cream adds lushness.

For stronger flavor, add two to three minced garlic cloves to the cauliflower before roasting. Another option is to sprinkle cauliflower with one teaspoon fresh thyme leaves and/or two tablespoons freshly grated Parmesan cheese during the last five to ten minutes of roasting.

To increase calories, use up to one cup heavy cream. If watching calories, omit cream altogether or substitute one-half cup low-fat milk.

Be very careful when blending soup in a blender or food processor. Let the soup cool slightly, don't fill the container more than two-thirds full, and secure the lid well before blending.

5 SERVINGS

1 large (about 2 pounds) head cauliflower, cut into large florets

1 to 2 tablespoons olive oil

Salt and freshly ground black pepper

3½ to 4 cups homemade chicken or vegetable broth (pages 40 or 74) or store-bought reduced-sodium broth

½ to 1 cup heavy cream

Preheat the oven to 425 degrees.

On a foil-lined, rimmed baking sheet, drizzle cauliflower with 1 tablespoon of the oil and toss to coat. Add the remaining 1 tablespoon of oil, if necessary. Sprinkle with salt and pepper. Roast for 25 to 35 minutes, or until very tender and slightly charred, tossing every 10 minutes.

Bring the broth to a boil and reduce the heat to a simmer. Transfer the cauliflower to a blender and add 3 ½ cups of the warmed broth and ½ cup of the cream. Blend until smooth, adding more broth or cream to achieve the desired consistency. (You may need to do this step in batches or transfer some of the mixture to a large bowl before adding all the liquid.)

PER SERVING	
Calories	140
Fat	12 g
Saturated fat	6 g
Cholesterol	30 mg
Sodium	370 mg
Carbohydrate	4 g
Dietary fiber	1 g
Sugars	2 g
Protein	4 g
Calcium	40 mg
Potassium	250 mg

TIP This recipe may not be suitable if you are experiencing gas or bloating.

Cantaloupe-Peach Soup

In warmer months, a chilled fruit soup is a lovely meal to celebrate what's in season. This soup really calls for a melon that is at the peak of its flavor, so make sure that your fruit is ripe and sweet.

A swirl of lightly sweetened sour cream is added before serving for a touch of creaminess. If you can tolerate the texture, add a sprinkle of fresh mint.

Load the blender in the order listed to make liquefying easier. If you are using a small blender, purée the cantaloupe in two batches so that it doesn't overwhelm the motor. If using frozen peaches, there's no need to defrost them first.

For a completely smooth soup, strain before serving.

4 SERVINGS

½ cup freshly squeezed or 100 percent orange juice

4 cups packed chopped cantaloupe or 1 cantaloupe, seeded and cut into 1-inch pieces

1 cup fresh or frozen peaches (peeled if fresh)

1 to 2 tablespoons fresh lime juice

1 tablespoon plus 2 teaspoons honey, divided use

Pinch salt

½ cup sour cream or plain Greek yogurt

¼ cup finely chopped fresh mint leaves, optional

In a blender, combine the orange juice and cantaloupe and process until smooth. Add the peaches, 1 tablespoon of the lime juice, 1 tablespoon of the honey, and salt and process until smooth, scraping down the sides to blend. Taste and add lime juice, if desired. Transfer to a bowl, cover, and refrigerate for 2 or more hours.

Before serving, combine the sour cream, the remaining 2 teaspoons of honey, and mint, if desired. Portion the soup into individual bowls and swirl a dollop of the sour cream into the soup.

PER SERVING	
Calories	170
Fat	5 g
Saturated fat	3.5 g
Cholesterol	20 mg
Sodium	80 mg
Carbohydrate	29 g
Dietary fiber	2 g
Sugars	26 g
Protein	3 g
Calcium	60 mg
Potassium	630 mg

TIP if you have a sore mouth or throat, omit the lime juice and substitute apple juice (or another of your choice) for the orange juice.

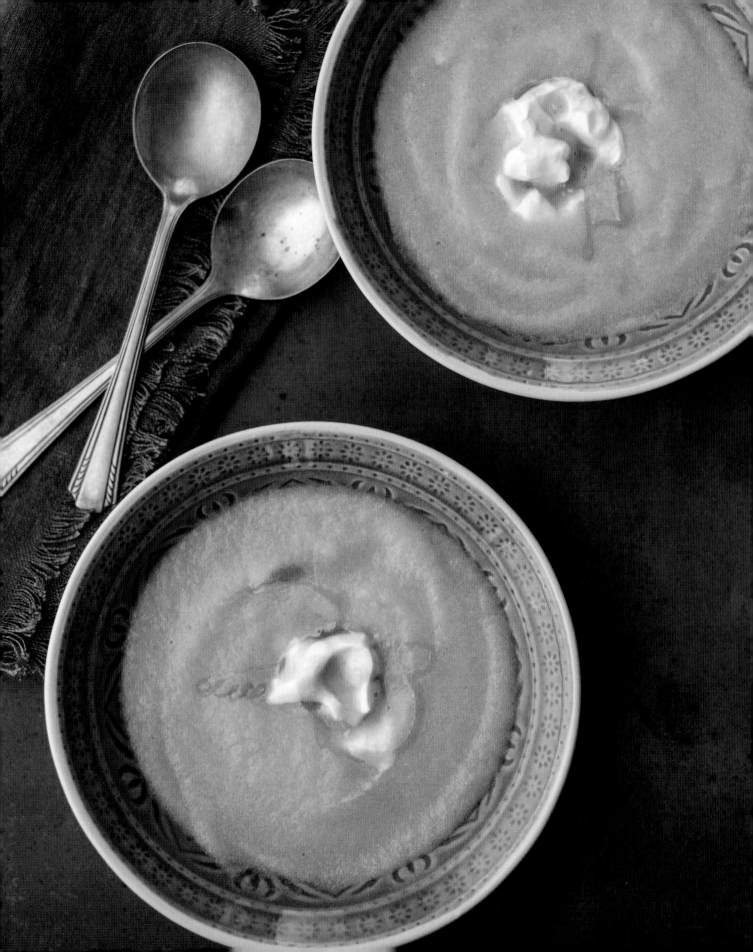

Sweet Potato and Cashew Purée

When it's hard to eat solid food, get needed nutrients from this vitamin A–rich vegetable purée fortified with cashews. Cashews add important plant-based fat, protein, and magnesium. This can also be made without the cashews. Make sure to cook them well to soften them if you have mouth sensitivity, or omit them.

Apple cider adds calories and a touch of sweetness without being overpowering. For food safety, be sure to use a bottled apple cider rather than a raw or unpasteurized variety.

2 SERVINGS

¼ cup finely chopped raw cashews

1 large sweet potato, peeled and cut into 1-inch pieces

½ to ¾ cup pasteurized apple cider or 100 percent apple juice

In a saucepan, cover the cashews with several inches of water and bring to a boil. Reduce the heat and simmer for 5 to 10 minutes. Add the sweet potatoes and simmer for 10 to 15 minutes, or until the potatoes and cashews are very tender. Strain the potato mixture and transfer the solids to a food processor. Add ½ cup of the apple cider and purée until smooth, scraping down the blade and sides to blend. If the purée is too thick, add apple cider a tablespoon at a time.

PER SERVING	
Calories	240
Fat	8 g
Saturated fat	1.5 g
Cholesterol	0 mg
Sodium	45 mg
Carbohydrate	39 g
Dietary fiber	5 g
Sugars	16 g
Protein	5 g
Calcium	50 mg
Potassium	530 mg

Mango Lassi

A lassi is a refreshing drink typically found in the Indian subcontinent. It contains yogurt and spices or fruit and comes in sweet, savory, and salty versions.

Using frozen mangos thickens the mixture and quickens the preparation by eliminating the need to peel and seed mangos. For easier blending, put the liquids and softer ingredients in the blender first.

If the mixture is too thick, dilute with additional milk. For a touch of acidity (if you don't have mouth sores), add a teaspoon or two of fresh lemon juice.

2 SERVINGS

¾ cup milk

¾ cup plain yogurt

2 tablespoons honey or agave syrup

1 cup frozen mango chunks

Pinch ground cinnamon

Pinch salt

In a blender, combine the milk, yogurt, honey, mango, cinnamon, and salt and blend until smooth.

PER SERVING

Calories	240
Fat	6 g
Saturated fat	3.5 g
Cholesterol	17 mg
Sodium	160 mg
Carbohydrate	42 g
Dietary fiber	1.5 g
Sugars	41 g
Protein	6 g
Calcium	230 mg
Potassium	440 mg

 TIP Traditionally, this drink is often topped with a sprinkle of chopped pistachios. When you're no longer having trouble swallowing or mouth tenderness, give it a try!

Cranberry-Lime Granita

A granita is a refreshing icy fruit treat, so elegant in appearance, it feels like a treat to eat. Its unique granular texture is achieved by frequently stirring the mixture while it freezes, which keeps the ice crystals small. This recipe is especially good if you have mouth tenderness, as chilled foods can soothe discomfort.

To limit the amount of sugar, use unsweetened cranberry juice, not cranberry cocktail. If you do not have mouth sores or irritation, add a tablespoon of lime juice before freezing for more tartness.

Once the mixture is fully icy, you can transfer it to a container and keep in the freezer until you are ready to eat it. If the mixture hardens too much, break it up in a food processor using the pulse feature.

14 SERVINGS

3 cups unsweetened cranberry juice, divided use

½ cup granulated sugar

Zest of 1 lime

In a small saucepan over medium heat, combine 1 cup of the cranberry juice and the sugar. Bring to a simmer, swirling the juice until the sugar completely dissolves.

Transfer to a 13-by-9-inch baking pan and let cool. Add the remaining 2 cups of cranberry juice and the lime zest. Freeze for 1 to 2 hours, or until the edges and bottom turn to ice. Using a fork, scrape the sides and bottom of the pan, and stir to redistribute. Return to the freezer and repeat every 30 to 60 minutes or until the mixture is uniformly icy.

PER SERVING	
Calories	50
Fat	0 g
Saturated fat	0 g
Cholesterol	0 mg
Sodium	0 mg
Carbohydrate	14 g
Dietary fiber	0 g
Sugars	14 g
Protein	0 g
Calcium	5 mg
Potassium	40 mg

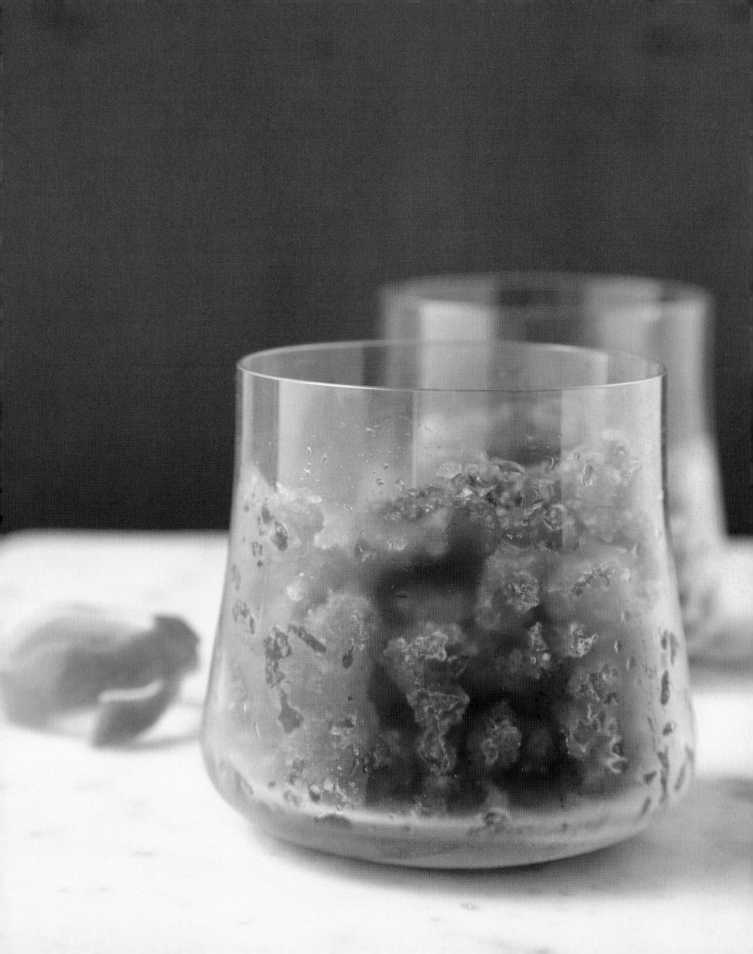

Vanilla Juice Glass Pudding

This mild, smooth-textured pudding will be welcome for someone having trouble swallowing or a sore mouth. For more sweetness, you can add another tablespoon of sugar. See page 179 for a refreshing strawberry version.

4 SERVINGS

1 (¼-ounce) package gelatin powder

¼ cup cold water

1 cup milk

½ cup granulated sugar

1 cup plain Greek yogurt

½ teaspoon vanilla extract

In a bowl, sprinkle the gelatin over the water and stir to dissolve. Set aside for 10 minutes.

Meanwhile, in a small saucepan over medium heat, combine the milk and the sugar. Bring to a simmer, swirling the milk until the sugar completely dissolves.

In a blender, combine the yogurt, vanilla, gelatin, and milk and process until smooth. Divide among four juice glasses. Refrigerate for 2 or more hours, or until firm.

PER SERVING

Calories	200
Fat	5 g
Saturated fat	2.5 g
Cholesterol	15 mg
Sodium	50 mg
Carbohydrate	30 g
Dietary fiber	0 g
Sugars	31 g
Protein	9 g
Calcium	130 mg
Potassium	160 mg

PB and Banana Smoothie

Who doesn't love the pairing of peanut butter and banana? Here those flavors combine for a thick, drinkable shake, perfect for a tender mouth. For easier blending, put the liquids and softer ingredients in the blender first. For extra sweetness, add a pitted Medjool date or two—just make sure to purée completely.

1 SERVING

¼ cup almond milk

¼ cup creamy peanut butter

½ to 1 cup ice cubes

1 ripe banana, cut into pieces

In a blender, combine the almond milk, banana, peanut butter, and ½ cup of the ice cubes and blend until smooth. For a colder and thinner shake, add more ice.

PER SERVING

Calories	500
Fat	34 g
Saturated fat	7 g
Cholesterol	0 mg
Sodium	340 mg
Carbohydrate	41 g
Dietary fiber	7 g
Sugars	21 g
Protein	18 g
Calcium	150 mg
Potassium	910 mg

TIP When bananas ripen before you are ready to use them, slice and freeze them in a zip-top bag to use in this and other smoothies and drinks or in Peanut Butter–Banana "Ice Cream" (page 180).

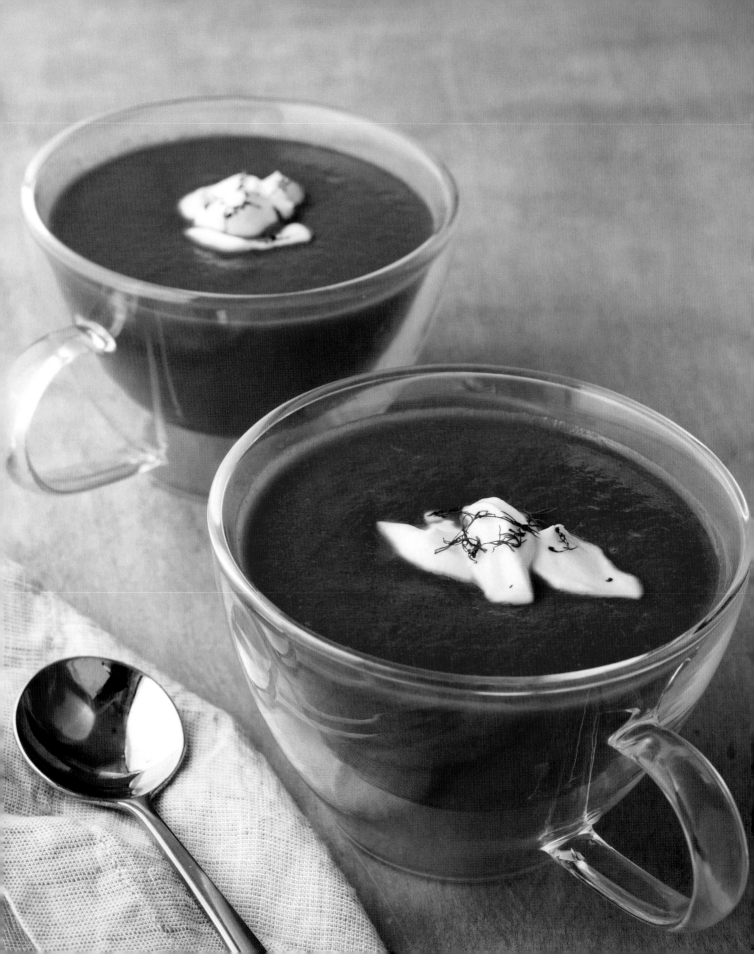

Chilled Beet Soup with Yogurt-Dill Swirl

Beets are a nutrient powerhouse, providing vitamin C, folate, fiber, and essential minerals like potassium and manganese.

After cooking, the skin of the beets should slip off easily, but beet juice can temporarily stain your hands and clothing. Use paper towels when peeling the beets to prevent this or run the beets under water while you remove the skin.

Make sure to allow a few hours for the soup to chill. Because the beets take an hour or more to cook, you can bake them early in the day or even the day before. Be careful opening the foil to check readiness, as there can be a lot of contained heat.

5 SERVINGS

1 1/2 pounds fresh beets, cut in half or quartered if large

1/4 cup balsamic vinegar, divided use

2 to 2 1/2 cups homemade chicken or vegetable broth (pages 40 or 74) or store-bought reduced-sodium broth

1 cup Greek yogurt, divided use

1 orange, juiced and zested (or 1/2 cup 100 percent orange juice)

2 tablespoons honey

1 tablespoon extra virgin olive oil

Salt and freshly ground black pepper

2 tablespoons finely chopped fresh dill

Preheat the oven to 400 degrees.

On a large sheet of heavy-duty aluminum foil, place the beets in a single layer and drizzle with 2 tablespoons of the balsamic vinegar. Wrap the foil around the beets, folding down the edges to seal well. Place the packet in the oven and bake for 1 to 1 1/2 hours, or until the beets are tender and easily pierced with a knife (use caution opening the foil). Set the packet aside to cool for 20 or more minutes.

Transfer the reserved cooking juices in the foil to a blender. Peel the skin off the beets and discard the skin. Cut the beets into large pieces and add to the blender. Add the remaining 2 tablespoons of balsamic vinegar, 2 cups of the broth, 1/2 cup of the yogurt, orange juice and zest, honey, and oil to the blender and process until smooth, scraping down the sides to blend. Season with salt and pepper. If the soup is too thick, add broth to desired consistency. Transfer to a bowl, cover, and refrigerate for 2 or more hours.

Before serving, combine the remaining 1/2 cup of yogurt and dill. Portion the soup into individual bowls and swirl a dollop of the yogurt into the soup.

PER SERVING	
Calories	160
Fat	6 g
Saturated fat	1.5 g
Cholesterol	10 mg
Sodium	280 mg
Carbohydrate	21 g
Dietary fiber	2 g
Sugars	19 g
Protein	7 g
Calcium	70 mg
Potassium	390 mg

Roasted Root Vegetable Soup

Using roasted vegetables takes much of the effort out of making homemade soup. Just spread the veggies on baking sheets and let the oven's heat transform them into creamy, soft, caramelized gems. Purée them with broth and the soup's on! Precise measurements aren't necessary; just add enough broth to make the soup as thick or thin as you can handle.

Depending on the size of your food processor, you might need to purée the vegetables in batches. If so, transfer the puréed mixture to a large bowl before adding all the broth.

Be careful when blending soups in a blender or food processor. Let the broth cool slightly, don't fill the container more than two-thirds full, and secure the lid well before blending.

7 SERVINGS

3 carrots, cut into 1-inch pieces

1 small (about 1 pound) butternut squash, peeled and seeded, cut into 1 1/4-inch pieces

1 small (about 8 ounces) sweet potato, peeled and cut into 1 1/4-inch pieces

1 small sweet or yellow onion, peeled and cut into 1 1/4-inch pieces

2 tablespoons olive oil

Salt and freshly ground black pepper

5 cups homemade chicken or vegetable broth (pages 40 or 74) or store-bought reduced-sodium broth

Preheat the oven to 400 degrees.

On two foil-lined, rimmed baking sheets, combine the carrots, squash, sweet potato, and onion. Drizzle with oil and toss to coat. Sprinkle with salt and pepper. Roast for 40 to 50 minutes, or until very tender and slightly charred, tossing every 15 minutes. Set aside.

Bring the broth to a boil and reduce heat to a simmer. Transfer the vegetables to a food processor and add 3 cups of the warmed broth. Blend until smooth, adding more of the broth to achieve the desired consistency. (You may need to do this step in batches or transfer the mixture to a large bowl before adding all the broth.)

PER SERVING

Calories	100
Fat	4.5 g
Saturated fat	0.5 g
Cholesterol	5 mg
Sodium	310 mg
Carbohydrate	12 g
Dietary fiber	3 g
Sugars	4 g
Protein	2 g
Calcium	40 mg
Potassium	320 mg

White Bean and Roasted Garlic Dip

Roasting garlic not only mellows its bitterness and adds depth of flavor, it also softens the cloves to a perfectly spreadable consistency. When added to a couple of cans of creamy white beans, you have a versatile dip or spread! This fiber- and protein-filled dip is a great option if you are looking for soft foods with a lot of flavor, and it can also be used as a vegetarian or vegan sandwich filling when swallowing problems have resolved.

If you are sensitive to citrus, start with one lemon and add more lemon juice to taste.

8 SERVINGS

10 garlic cloves, peeled

¼ cup extra virgin olive oil

1 (15-ounce) can navy beans, rinsed and drained

1 (15-ounce) can cannellini beans, rinsed and drained

Juice of 2 lemons

½ to 1 teaspoon salt

Pinch or 2 cayenne pepper

Preheat the oven to 400 degrees.

In a ramekin or small baking pan, combine the garlic and olive oil. Cover with foil and bake for 20 to 30 minutes, or until the garlic is golden and soft. Set aside to cool.

In a food processor, combine the garlic and olive oil, both beans, lemon juice, ½ teaspoon of the salt, and a pinch of the cayenne and process until smooth, scraping down the blade and sides to blend. Taste and add salt or cayenne, if desired. Store unused dip in a covered container in the refrigerator.

PER SERVING	
Calories	150
Fat	7 g
Saturated fat	1 g
Cholesterol	0 mg
Sodium	240 mg
Carbohydrate	17 g
Dietary fiber	5 g
Sugars	0.5 g
Protein	5 g
Calcium	40 mg
Potassium	260 mg

Love Your Greens Shake

When making vegetable or fruit shakes, one of the advantages of using a blender instead of a juicer is that all the nutrients and fiber stay in the drink instead of being extracted as pulp. This recipe, made with a variety of vitamin-rich hearty greens and fresh fruit, will work best using a high-powered blender, such as a Vitamix.

For better blending, most manufacturers suggest adding liquids first so that they are closest to the blade. Then add ingredients from softest to most dense, and ice cubes last. Check your blender's instructions for the best order for your machine.

Feel free to swap out ingredients with whatever fruits and veggies you have on hand. Half the fun is experimenting! Just be sure to wash your greens well before using.

2 SERVINGS

½ cup water

Juice of ½ lemon

½ avocado, peeled and pitted

1 cup fresh spinach leaves

1 cup kale leaves, thick ribs removed

1 apple, cored and quartered

1 cup seedless green grapes, chopped pineapple, or chopped mango

2 tablespoons coarsely chopped mint leaves

1 cup ice cubes

In a high-powered blender, combine the water, lemon juice, avocado, spinach, kale, apple, grapes, mint, and ice cubes. Start on low and increase to high speed for about 1 minute, or until smooth.

PER SERVING

Calories	160
Fat	6 g
Saturated fat	1 g
Cholesterol	0 mg
Sodium	30 mg
Carbohydrate	30 g
Dietary fiber	6 g
Sugars	20 g
Protein	2 g
Calcium	60 mg
Potassium	560 mg

TIP If you have mouth or throat pain, omit the lemon juice and don't prepare the drink with pineapple—both can make mouth tenderness worse.

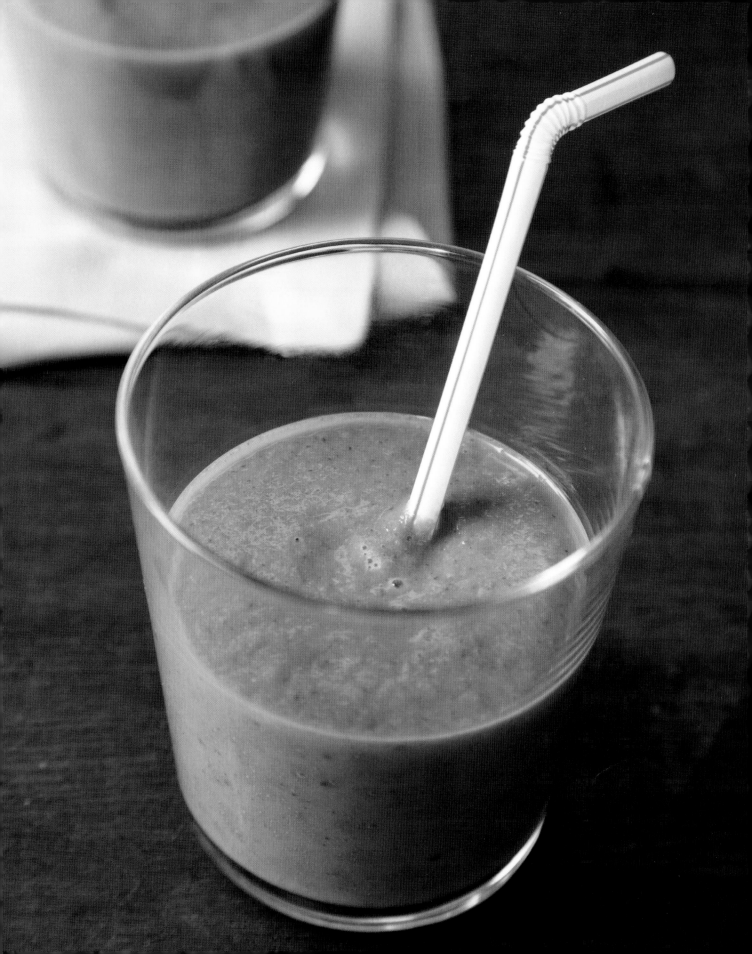

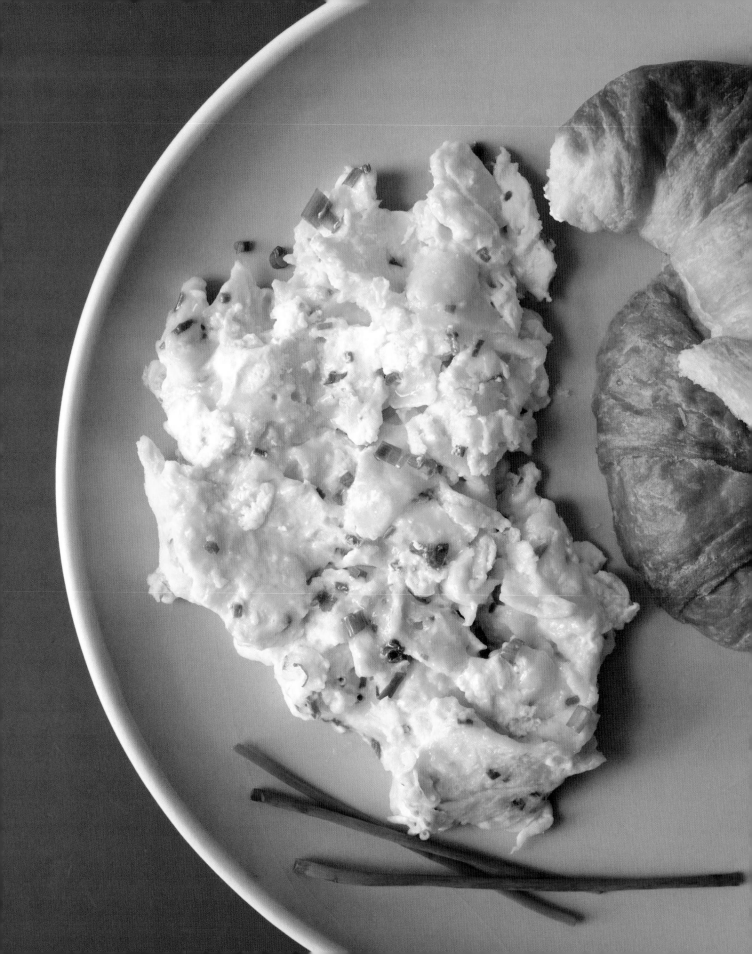

SM SORE MOUTH OR THROAT

Blueberry-Cottage Cheese Pancakes

Slow Cooker Split Pea and Potato Soup

Chocolate-Peanut Butter Balls

Bread Pudding with Butternut Squash, Mushrooms, and Spinach

Overnight Refrigerator Oats with Peaches and Honey

Hummus-Egg Salad

Raspberry- and Cream Cheese-Stuffed French Toast

Creamy Polenta

Carrot-Ginger Soup

Scrambled Eggs with Cream Cheese and Chives

Slow-Cooked Oatmeal

Fruity Yogurt Bark

Fresh Strawberry Juice Glass Pudding

Peanut Butter-Banana "Ice Cream"

Noodle Kugel

Farro "Risotto" with Chicken, Portobellos, and Spinach

Rosemary-White Bean Soup

Mini Chicken Pot Pies

Simple Herb Risotto

CANCER TREATMENT CAN CAUSE SOME PEOPLE TO DEVELOP A SORE MOUTH AND/OR THROAT. Certain chemotherapy medications can cause these symptoms, as can radiation therapy to the head and neck area or to the esophagus. Sore mouth as related to treatment is known as mucositis, and if the throat is affected, it is known as esophagitis. For someone dealing with this side effect, the mouth, tongue, gums, or throat can appear red, shiny, or even swollen. Sometimes small sores or ulcers can occur. When cancer treatment has finished, your mouth and throat will heal.

Regular rinsing throughout the day with a homemade mouth rinse will help to keep your mouth clean, promote healing, and even help foods taste better. Simply mix together four cups of water, one teaspoon of salt, and one teaspoon of baking soda. Swish the mixture in your mouth and spit out.

Mucositis, oral sores, or esophagitis can make eating painful, and your favorite foods may irritate your mouth or throat. If you are having pain that interferes with eating, ask your doctor about medication to relieve the pain and discomfort you feel with chewing and swallowing. Some medicines can be swished in the mouth before meals or sipped on to coat the mouth and throat, and there are others that can be applied to painful areas.

If you are having these problems, soft or semisoft, bland, room-temperature foods will likely be easier to chew and swallow. These suggestions may help:

- Avoid rough-textured foods, such as dry toast, crackers, pretzels, granola, raw vegetables and fruits, or fried or baked foods with rough exteriors or coatings.

- Eat soft foods, such as cream-based soups, mashed potatoes, yogurt, scrambled eggs, custards, puddings, cooked cereals, ice cream, and milk shakes. Other soft foods that may work include noodles, casseroles, cottage cheese, gelatin, applesauce, or canned fruit.

- Moisten dry foods with broth, gravy, or sauces.

- Choose lukewarm or cool foods. Very hot foods can cause discomfort. Some people find cool or even icy foods to be soothing.

- Avoid tart, acidic, or salty foods and drinks, such as citrus fruits (grapefruit, orange, lemon, or lime), certain tropical fruits (pineapple, papaya, or kiwi), pickled and vinegar-based foods, and tomato-based foods and drinks.

- Blend, purée, or liquefy foods in a blender or food processor to make them easier to eat. Add enough liquid (broth, juice, or milk) to achieve the desired consistency.

- Avoid tobacco products and commercial mouthwashes that contain alcohol.

CONTACT YOUR DOCTOR IN THESE SITUATIONS:

- Your mouth or throat is sore or inflamed.

- You have open sores or ulcers in your mouth.

- Your gums are bleeding.

- There are white patches on your tongue or on the inside of your mouth.

For more information about managing a sore mouth or throat, visit the American Cancer Society website at cancer.org or call 800-227-2345.

Blueberry–Cottage Cheese Pancakes

Cottage cheese adds protein and an airy quality to these griddlecakes, which are easy on the mouth and the stomach and taste good any time of day. Cottage cheese not only provides calcium, it contains more protein per ounce than Greek yogurt.

To prevent the pancakes from sticking, make sure your skillet is hot before adding the batter. Do the flick test: flick a drop of water onto the pan before adding the batter. It should sizzle. Although you want a hot pan initially, monitor the heat once the pancakes are on to make sure they don't cook too quickly. Peek at the bottoms to make sure they are turning an even golden color and not browning too fast. If they are, reduce the heat and continue to watch them to know when to flip them. You want the pancakes to be golden brown and firm to make turning them easier.

Serve plain, with maple syrup, or topped with a blueberry or fruit compote.

8 PANCAKES

1/3 cup all-purpose flour	1/4 teaspoon salt	1/2 cup milk
1/3 cup whole wheat flour	1/2 cup fresh or frozen blueberries, defrosted	1 tablespoon canola oil
2 tablespoons granulated sugar		1/2 teaspoon vanilla extract
1 teaspoon baking powder	2 eggs	1/2 cup cottage cheese

In a bowl, combine both flours, sugar, baking powder, and salt. Add the blueberries and stir to coat with flour. Set aside.

In a bowl, beat the eggs. Add the milk, oil, and vanilla and stir to combine. Add the cottage cheese and stir to combine. Add mixture to the dry ingredients and gently stir until just combined.

Coat a griddle or skillet with nonstick cooking spray and preheat over medium heat. Spoon 1/4 cup of batter, spacing them 3 to 4 inches apart. You should be able to fit several at a time. Cook for 1 minute or until the pancakes are golden brown on the bottom and bubbly on top.

Carefully flip the pancakes and cook for 1 to 2 minutes, or until cooked through. Repeat with remaining batter.

PER SERVING
(ONE PANCAKE)

Calories	110
Fat	4 g
Saturated fat	1 g
Cholesterol	50 mg
Sodium	190 mg
Carbohydrate	13 g
Dietary fiber	1 g
Sugars	5 g
Protein	5 g
Calcium	80 mg
Potassium	90 mg

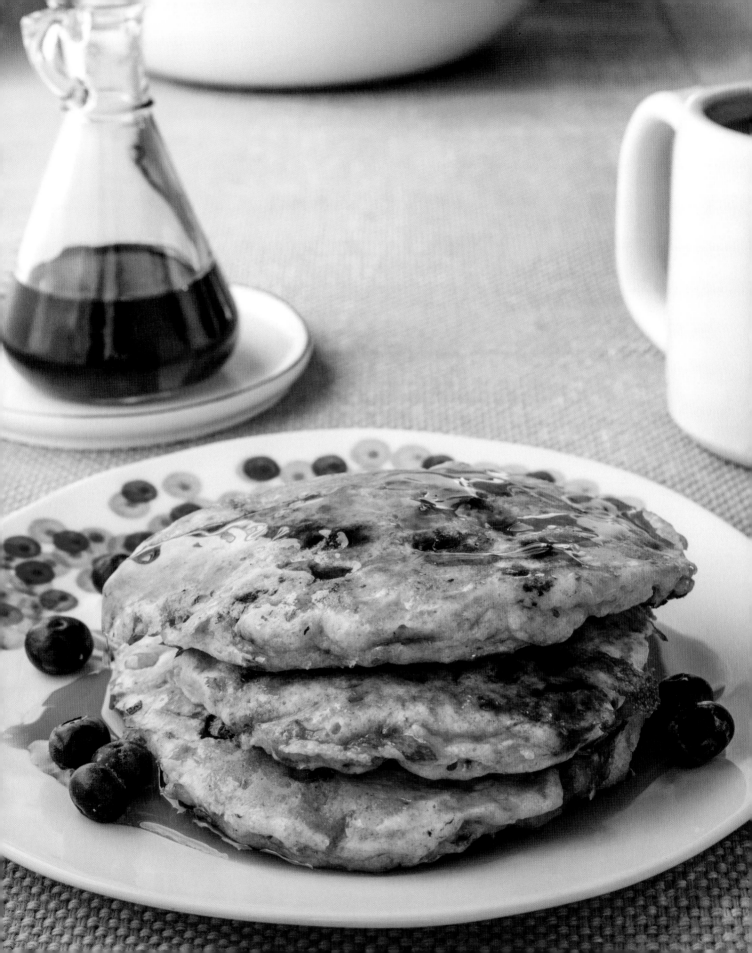

Slow Cooker Split Pea and Potato Soup

This wholesome soup, rich with heart-healthy legumes and veggies, feels substantial even though it goes down easy. If swallowing isn't an issue, leave tender pieces of carrot or potato in the soup; if you have difficulty swallowing, purée the soup before serving. If the soup is too thick, add broth or water.

If you don't have an immersion blender, transfer a few cups of soup to the blender at a time and purée. Be very careful when puréeing soup in a blender or food processor. Let the soup cool slightly, don't fill the container more than two-thirds full, and secure the lid well before blending.

7 SERVINGS

4 cups homemade chicken or vegetable broth (pages 40 or 74) or store-bought reduced-sodium broth

1 cup dried split peas

2 carrots, sliced

1 russet potato, peeled and cut into 1-inch pieces

1 onion, coarsely chopped

1 celery stalk, sliced

2 fresh thyme sprigs or 1 teaspoon dried thyme

1 to 2 teaspoons salt

In a slow cooker, combine the broth, split peas, carrots, potato, onion, celery, thyme, and 1 teaspoon of the salt and cook on high for 4 to 5 hours or on low for 6 to 8 hours, or until the peas and vegetables are very tender. Discard the thyme sprigs. With an immersion blender, partially purée the soup, leaving some pieces of vegetables whole, as desired. Season with additional salt, if desired.

PER SERVING

Calories	130
Fat	1 g
Saturated fat	0 g
Cholesterol	5 mg
Sodium	640 mg
Carbohydrate	24 g
Dietary fiber	8 g
Sugars	4 g
Protein	8 g
Calcium	30 mg
Potassium	460 mg

 TIP This soup can also be made on the stovetop.

Chocolate–Peanut Butter Balls

Nonfat dry milk firms up these confections while providing extra calcium in addition to protein. Unlike other peanut butter balls, which are laden with powdered sugar or corn syrup, these four-ingredient snacks aren't overly sweet, making them good for snacking.

If using unsweetened natural peanut butter, you might need to add a little more honey.

10 SERVINGS

¹/₂ cup smooth peanut butter

¹/₃ to ¹/₂ cup nonfat dry milk

3 tablespoons honey

2 tablespoons unsweetened cocoa powder

In a bowl, combine the peanut butter, ¹/₃ cup of the nonfat dry milk, honey, and cocoa powder. If necessary, add dry milk, a tablespoon at a time, until the mixture is no longer overly sticky. Roll the mixture into ten golf ball–sized portions. Refrigerate until ready to eat.

PER SERVING (ONE BALL)

Calories	110
Fat	7 g
Saturated fat	1.5 g
Cholesterol	0 mg
Sodium	70 mg
Carbohydrate	10 g
Dietary fiber	1 g
Sugars	8 g
Protein	4 g
Calcium	40 mg
Potassium	140 mg

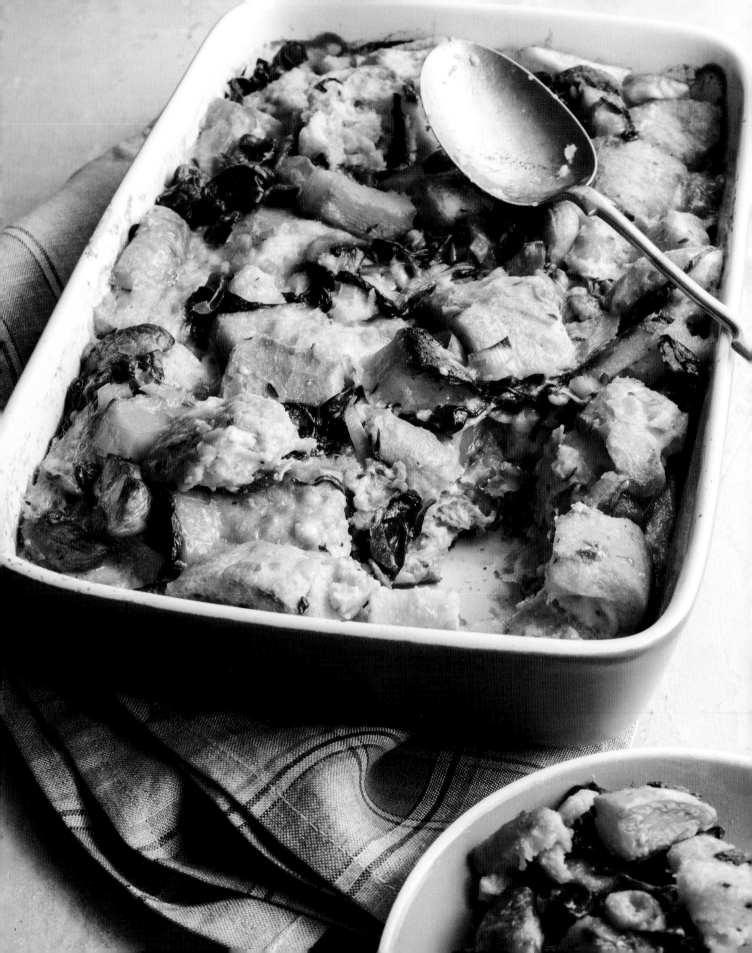

Bread Pudding with Butternut Squash, Mushrooms, and Spinach

This mild, stuffing-type dish can be served as a vegetarian entrée or a side with a protein. Use a thinner-crusted ciabatta or baguette, rather than a heartier bread, to ensure a softer finished dish.

8 TO 10 SERVINGS

1 medium butternut squash, peeled, seeded, and cut into 3/4-inch cubes

2 tablespoons olive oil, divided use

Salt

4 eggs

2 cups milk

1 packed cup (4 ounces) grated Gruyère cheese

1/2 cup freshly grated Parmesan cheese

8 ounces stale bread, cut into 1-inch cubes

1 leek, white and light green parts only, sliced

8 ounces white mushrooms, sliced

2 garlic cloves, minced

1 teaspoon dried thyme

1 (5- to 6-ounce) package fresh baby spinach

Freshly ground black pepper

Preheat the oven to 425 degrees. Lightly coat a rimmed baking sheet with nonstick cooking spray. Top with the squash. Drizzle with 1 tablespoon of the oil, sprinkle with salt, and stir to combine. Evenly distribute the squash on the baking sheet. Bake for 20 to 30 minutes, or until tender and slightly charred, stirring the squash every 10 minutes.

Meanwhile, in a large bowl, beat the eggs and milk. Add both cheeses and the bread cubes and stir to combine. Set the mixture aside, pushing the bread down occasionally, so that it absorbs the liquid.

In a large skillet over medium-high heat, add the remaining 1 tablespoon of oil. Sauté the leek for 5 minutes. Add the mushrooms and sauté until softened. Add the garlic and thyme and sauté for 1 minute. Stir in the spinach,

a handful at a time, and sauté until wilted. Season with salt and pepper.

When the squash is done cooking, reduce the oven temperature to 375 degrees. Add the squash and the mushroom mixture to the bread and stir to combine. Lightly coat a 9-by-13-inch (or other 2-quart) baking pan with nonstick cooking spray. Transfer the mixture to the prepared baking pan and cover with foil.

Bake for 30 minutes. Remove the foil and bake for 10 minutes, or until puffed and golden brown.

PER SERVING

Calories	290
Fat	15 g
Saturated fat	6 g
Cholesterol	120 mg
Sodium	390 mg
Carbohydrate	26 g
Dietary fiber	3 g
Sugars	7 g
Protein	15 g
Calcium	370 mg
Potassium	510 mg

Overnight Refrigerator Oats with Peaches and Honey

Refrigerator oats are a refreshing way to start your day and are easy on a tender mouth. They are similar to muesli (an oat, nut, and dried fruit mixture soaked in liquid overnight to soften). Since this version is intended for those with mouth sensitivity, dried fruit, nuts, and seeds are omitted, but feel free to include them once you are feeling up to it. For a thicker and creamier mixture, fold in Greek yogurt to individual portions, if desired.

Either fresh or frozen peaches can be used. You should be able to chop the peaches while they are still frozen, but if not, partially defrost them until they cut more easily. Their juices will flavor the mixture as it chills overnight. If you're using fresh peaches, peel them first.

4 SERVINGS

2 cups old-fashioned rolled oats

1 1/4 cups chopped fresh or frozen peaches, defrosted

Pinch salt

Pinch or 2 ground cinnamon

2 cups almond milk, soy milk, or milk

1 tablespoon honey or agave syrup

In a bowl, combine the oats, peaches, salt, and cinnamon. Add the milk and honey and stir to combine. Cover and refrigerate overnight. Before serving, portion the oats into individual bowls.

PER SERVING

Calories	210
Fat	4 g
Saturated fat	0.5 g
Cholesterol	0 mg
Sodium	130 mg
Carbohydrate	37 g
Dietary fiber	5 g
Sugars	9 g
Protein	6 g
Calcium	250 mg
Potassium	330 mg

Hummus-Egg Salad

Instead of using mayonnaise to bind boiled eggs for egg salad, why not use protein-rich hummus? Not only does it hold the mixture together, making it good if you are having problems swallowing, it also adds a subtle nuttiness. Some finely chopped fresh dill adds brightness.

1 SERVING

1 hard-boiled egg, finely chopped

¼ cup prepared plain hummus

1 teaspoon finely chopped fresh dill

Salt

In a bowl, combine the egg, hummus, and dill. Season with salt.

PER SERVING	
Calories	180
Fat	11 g
Saturated fat	2.5 g
Cholesterol	185 mg
Sodium	310 mg
Carbohydrate	9 g
Dietary fiber	4 g
Sugars	4 g
Protein	11 g
Calcium	50 mg
Potassium	210 mg

TIP For the family (or when the side effect has resolved), season with freshly ground black pepper to taste.

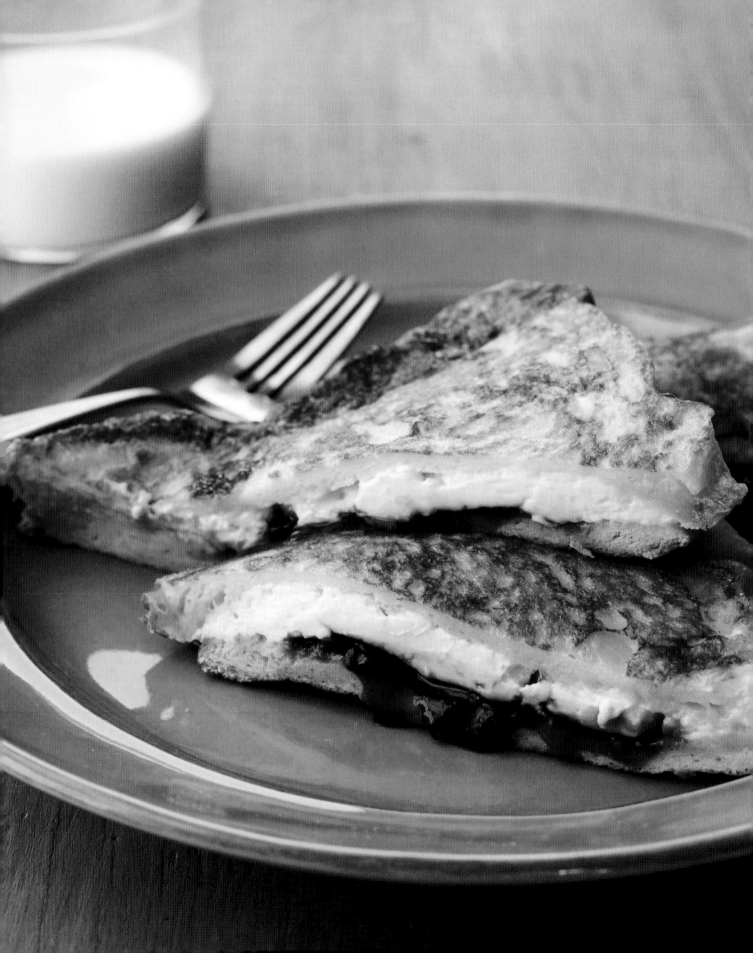

Raspberry- and Cream Cheese–Stuffed French Toast

Here, melt-in-your-mouth French toast holds a delicious surprise: a filling of cream cheese and jam. This sumptuous "sandwich," made with a soft egg-soaked bread such as challah or brioche, is especially good for sensitive mouths.

You can substitute a nut butter, ricotta, Greek yogurt, or cottage cheese for the cream cheese and use any seedless jam or even honey.

2 SERVINGS

1 egg

⅓ cup whole milk

½ teaspoon vanilla extract

2 (1-inch thick) slices challah, brioche, or soft white bread

2 tablespoons whipped or softened cream cheese

4 teaspoons seedless raspberry, blueberry, or other jam

½ teaspoon butter

In a shallow bowl, beat the egg. Add the milk and vanilla and whisk to combine.

Cut each slice of bread ¾ of the way through. Gently open the sides, as if you were opening a book. Spread 1 tablespoon of cream cheese on one side of the inside of the bread. Spread 2 teaspoons of jam on top of the cream cheese. "Close" the sides of the bread, pressing down to adhere. Repeat with the other slice.

Place one piece of bread at a time in the egg mixture and turn to coat several times.

In a skillet or griddle over medium heat, melt the butter. Carefully place both pieces of bread in the skillet and cook until the bottoms are golden brown. Carefully flip and cook until the other side is golden brown, pressing down with the spatula occasionally.

PER SERVING	
Calories	380
Fat	15 g
Saturated fat	6 g
Cholesterol	155 mg
Sodium	500 mg
Carbohydrate	50 g
Dietary fiber	2 g
Sugars	10 g
Protein	13 g
Calcium	110 mg
Potassium	210 mg

TIP Use leftover cream cheese for the Scrambled Eggs with Cream Cheese and Chives (page 175) or Spinach–Artichoke Dip Quesadillas (page 199).

Creamy Polenta

Polenta, slowly cooked cornmeal, is easy on the mouth and stomach. The longer it cooks, the more complex the flavors become. This unorthodox method of mixing the cornmeal with the water before heating it (instead of the more typical technique of adding the cornmeal to boiling water) guarantees splatter-free cooking and a smooth end result.

You can make a more calorie-dense dish by adding one cup of grated or shredded cheese during the last minute of cooking or substituting milk for the water.

If very soft polenta is desired, thin it with added water, milk, or cream. For a firmer polenta, transfer the cooked polenta to a baking pan and it will firm up as it sits. To reheat soft polenta, add a little water to the mixture to smooth it out while heating.

4 TO 6 SERVINGS

4 cups water

1 cup cornmeal

1 teaspoon salt

1 tablespoon butter

In a saucepan off the heat, combine the water, cornmeal, and salt until smooth. Place over medium heat and bring to a boil, whisking constantly. Reduce the heat to low and cook for 40 to 45 minutes, stirring frequently, scraping down the sides and the bottom of the pan to prevent sticking and burning. Stir in the butter until totally melted.

PER SERVING

Calories	150
Fat	3.5 g
Saturated fat	2 g
Cholesterol	8 mg
Sodium	520 mg
Carbohydrate	27 g
Dietary fiber	1 g
Sugars	1 g
Protein	3 g
Calcium	10 mg
Potassium	50 mg

TIP Polenta doesn't have to be a savory dish only. If you are craving something sweeter, use the polenta as a variation on oatmeal and top with a fruit compote or fresh berries and drizzle with honey.

Carrot-Ginger Soup

Using a food processor to chop the vegetables makes the prep time super quick for this soup. Use quick pulses just until the onion is chopped to prevent it from getting mushy. Once you've started cooking the onion, chop the carrots. There's no need to worry about getting the sizes just right since the soup is puréed after cooking.

The cream adds richness and calories. For a milder soup, reduce or eliminate the amount of ginger.

Be very careful when blending soup in a blender or food processor. Let the soup cool slightly, don't fill the container more than two-thirds full, and secure the lid well before blending.

5 SERVINGS

2 garlic cloves

1 (1 ¼-inch) piece fresh ginger, peeled

1 onion, quartered

2 tablespoons butter or canola oil

1 pound carrots, cut into 1- to 2-inch pieces, or a 1-pound bag baby carrots, rinsed

4 cups homemade chicken broth (page 40) or store-bought reduced-sodium broth

½ cup heavy cream, optional

Salt and freshly ground black pepper

In a food processor, with the motor running, drop in the garlic and ginger and purée. Stop the machine, add the onion, and pulse until evenly chopped.

In a stockpot over medium heat, melt the butter. Sauté the onion mixture for 5 to 8 minutes, or until softened.

Meanwhile, pulse the carrots in the food processor until finely chopped. Add to the onion mixture and sauté for 3 to 5 minutes. Add the broth and stir to combine. Bring to a boil. Reduce the heat, partially cover, and simmer for 30 to 40 minutes, or until very tender, stirring occasionally. Stir in the cream, if desired. Cool slightly.

Transfer to a blender or food processor and purée (you may need to do this step in two or more batches). Season with salt and pepper.

PER SERVING	
Calories	100
Fat	6 g
Saturated fat	3 g
Cholesterol	15 mg
Sodium	490 mg
Carbohydrate	12 g
Dietary fiber	3 g
Sugars	5 g
Protein	3 g
Calcium	40 mg
Potassium	330 mg

 TIP Add calories by increasing the amount of cream used to 1 cup. If you are trying to lose weight, omit the cream.

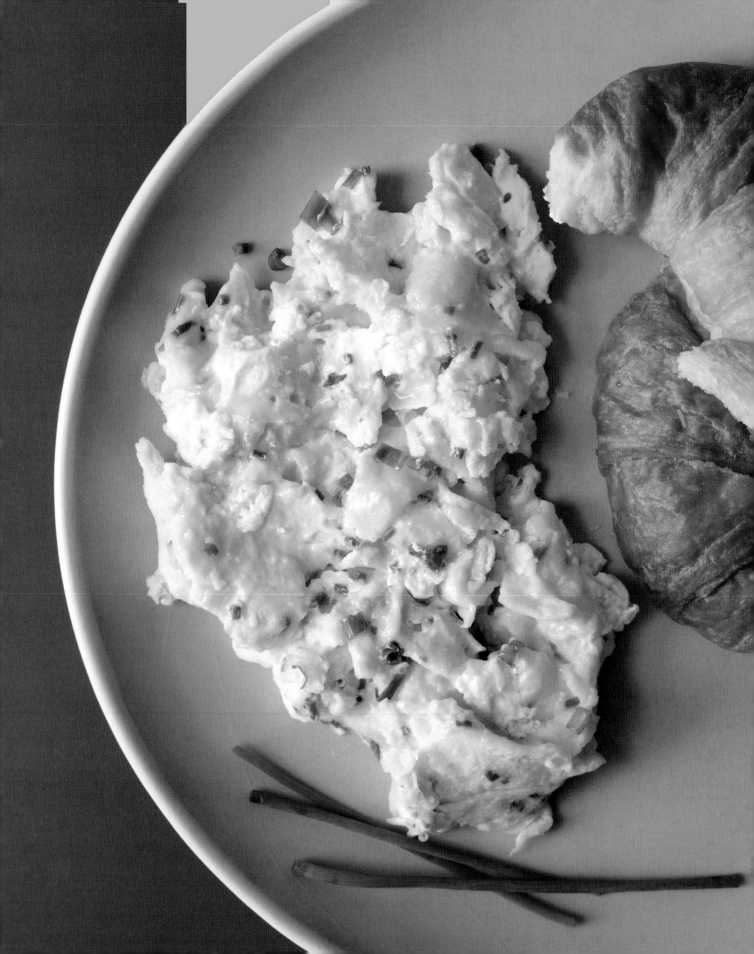

Scrambled Eggs with Cream Cheese and Chives

Eggs are so versatile and can be eaten virtually any time of day. When you are looking to add calories and feel indulged, this pairing of eggs and cream cheese satisfies hunger with a lush mouth-feel. A sprinkle of chives makes it sing.

If your mouth is very tender, omit the chives. If you are having trouble swallowing, make sure the eggs are softly scrambled.

2 SERVINGS

1 teaspoon butter or olive oil

4 eggs, beaten

2 tablespoons cream cheese, cut into ½-inch pieces

1 tablespoon thinly sliced chives

In an 8- or 10-inch, preferably nonstick, skillet, over medium heat, melt the butter, swirling it to coat the bottom of the pan. Add the eggs and cook without stirring for 10 seconds. Top with cream cheese, distributing it evenly over the eggs, and sprinkle with chives. Using a spatula, gently stir to combine the eggs and cream cheese, until the eggs are cooked through.

PER SERVING

Calories	210
Fat	16 g
Saturated fat	7 g
Cholesterol	395 mg
Sodium	200 mg
Carbohydrate	1 g
Dietary fiber	0 g
Sugars	1 g
Protein	14 g
Calcium	70 mg
Potassium	160 mg

Slow-Cooked Oatmeal

Steel-cut oats are made with the whole groat, which provides more nutrients and a toothsome texture. This heartier variety takes longer to cook, so using a slow cooker frees you from being tied to the stove during cooking. As good as this oatmeal is the first day, it holds up on the second day as well. Keep any uneaten oatmeal in the refrigerator and thin it with milk or water before reheating it.

The time to prepare this dish might vary a bit depending on your equipment and the consistency that you prefer your oatmeal. If you are unsure about your slow cooker, try it during the day so that you can gauge how long it takes, tasting the oatmeal after two to three hours and comparing it to seven hours, the equivalent of all night.

For a thicker, creamier oatmeal (and extra protein and calcium), stir in nonfat dry milk after cooking, or if the oatmeal is thicker than you'd like, dilute it with regular milk. Other options for added protein include stirring in creamy peanut or almond butter, Greek yogurt, or cottage cheese.

4 SERVINGS

4 cups water

1 cup steel-cut oats

1/2 teaspoon salt

1/2 teaspoon vanilla extract

1/2 teaspoon ground cinnamon

1/2 cup nonfat dry milk, Fortified Milk (page 194), or regular milk, optional

Brown sugar, maple syrup, sliced banana, blueberries, optional

Generously coat the inside of a slow cooker with nonstick cooking spray. Add the water, oats, salt, vanilla, and cinnamon. Stir to combine, cover, and cook on low for 3 to 7 hours. If the oatmeal sets around the edges, scrape it off and mix into the softer middle.

When ready to eat, add nonfat dry milk, Fortified Milk, or regular milk a tablespoon at a time, if desired, until it reaches the consistency you prefer. Portion into individual bowls and add toppings, if desired.

PER SERVING	
Calories	140
Fat	2.5 g
Saturated fat	0.5 g
Cholesterol	0 mg
Sodium	300 mg
Carbohydrate	27 g
Dietary fiber	4 g
Sugars	0 g
Protein	6 g
Calcium	30 mg
Potassium	170 mg

TIP For the family (or when the side effect has resolved), add raisins, chopped dried figs, chopped walnuts or almonds, or toasted coconut in addition to the mix-ins listed above.

Fruity Yogurt Bark

This homemade frozen yogurt bark is ideal when you want something sweet to suck or nibble on for relief. Slightly sweetened, protein-rich Greek yogurt is mixed with fruit purée for a creamy chilled treat. Letting the fruit macerate first produces a syrupy mixture that blends easily into the yogurt, flavoring it throughout. You can also add plain chopped fresh fruit or berries into the honey-sweetened yogurt mixture for more pronounced flavor and different textures.

Use your favorite fruit or berry or a combination (packages of frozen assorted berries are handy to keep in your freezer for this and for the Strawberry-Blueberry "Mocktail" on page 228).

If room is tight in your freezer, use a small rimmed sheet, like one used in a toaster oven.

Hold the pieces with parchment paper or a napkin for easy eating.

8 SERVINGS

1 cup fresh or frozen blueberries, defrosted

1 tablespoon granulated sugar

1 cup plain Greek yogurt

1 to 2 tablespoons honey

1/2 teaspoon vanilla extract

Pinch salt

Line a small, rimmed baking sheet with parchment paper.

In a bowl, combine the berries and sugar. Set aside for 15 to 30 minutes, or until the berries soften and juices form. Transfer to a blender and blend until smooth. Strain the mixture through a fine mesh sieve into a container or bowl, pushing down with a spoon to extract all the liquid. Add the yogurt, 1 tablespoon of the honey, vanilla, and salt and stir to combine. Taste and add honey, if desired.

Pour into the center of the prepared sheet and spread 1/4-inch thick. Freeze for 3 or more hours, or until firm. Break into pieces to serve.

PER SERVING	
Calories	45
Fat	1.5 g
Saturated fat	0.5 g
Cholesterol	4 mg
Sodium	25 mg
Carbohydrate	5 g
Dietary fiber	0 g
Sugars	5 g
Protein	3 g
Calcium	30 mg
Potassium	40 mg

TIP For the family (or when the side effect has resolved), mash the fruit instead of blending it to keep some pieces of fruit in the bark. You can also top the mixture with chopped pistachios or almonds or toasted coconut before freezing for added texture and flavor. With these additions, this recipe would also be good for constipation.

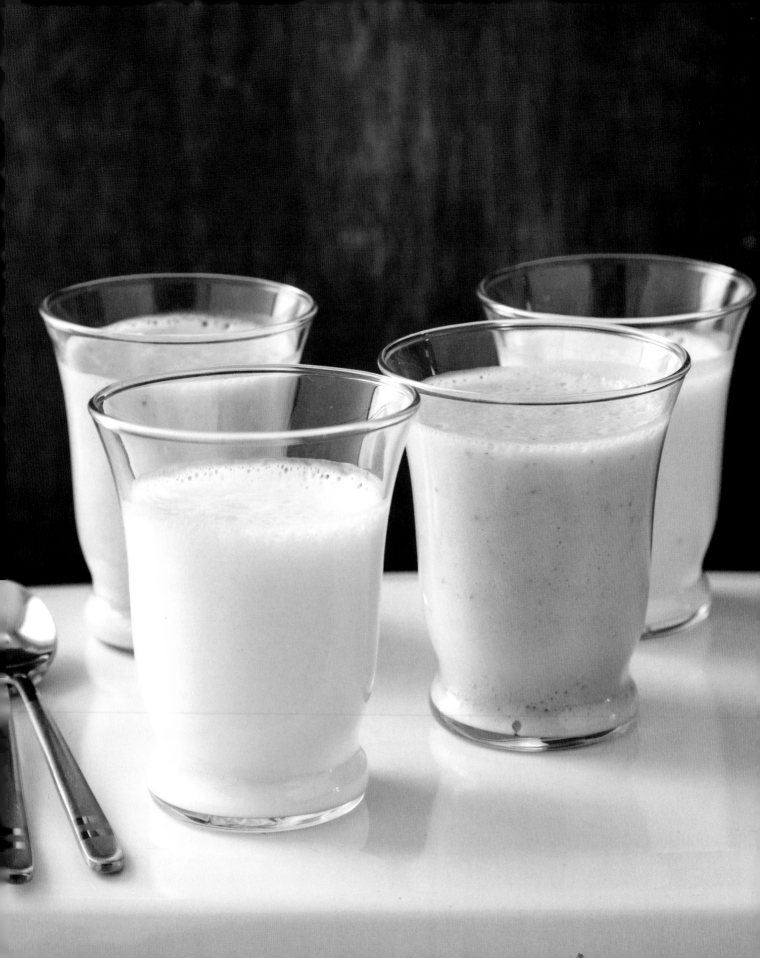

Fresh Strawberry Juice Glass Pudding

This simple pudding, thickened with unflavored gelatin, is good to have on hand for when you want something comforting with a hint of sweetness. Divide the mixture into juice glasses for perfect portioning. You can substitute another fruit for the macerated strawberries if desired. If you crave something sweeter, add another tablespoon of sugar.

For a vanilla version of this pudding (also pictured), see page 150.

6 SERVINGS

2 cups sliced fresh strawberries

2 tablespoons plus ½ cup granulated sugar, divided use

1 (¼-ounce) package gelatin powder

¼ cup cold water

1 cup milk

1 cup plain Greek yogurt

In a bowl, combine the strawberries and 2 tablespoons of the sugar. Set aside for 20 minutes, or until the strawberries soften and juices form.

Meanwhile, in a bowl, sprinkle the gelatin over the water and stir to dissolve. Set aside for 10 minutes.

In a small saucepan over medium heat, combine the milk and the remaining ½ cup of sugar. Bring to a simmer, swirling the milk until the sugar completely dissolves.

In a blender, combine the yogurt, strawberries and their juice, gelatin, and milk and process until smooth. Divide among six juice glasses. Refrigerate for 2 or more hours, or until firm.

PER SERVING	
Calories	160
Fat	3.5 g
Saturated fat	1.5 g
Cholesterol	9 mg
Sodium	35 mg
Carbohydrate	29 g
Dietary fiber	1 g
Sugars	27 g
Protein	6 g
Calcium	90 mg
Potassium	190 mg

Peanut Butter–Banana "Ice Cream"

When you find yourself with extra ripe bananas, slice and freeze them to use later in smoothies or in this delicious, creamy, and rich ice cream-like frosty treat, made with only two ingredients. It doesn't get much easier than this!

Make sure your banana is ripe enough to eat as is but not overly mushy. A sturdy food processor works best. Don't worry if it makes a few clunking noises when you start processing. The bananas will seem powdery at first and then form a softer mass with extra creamy purée around the sides of the bowl.

For a real indulgence, drizzle with chocolate syrup before serving.

1 SERVING

1 small ripe banana, sliced

1 tablespoon creamy peanut butter

Place the banana slices on a wax paper- or parchment paper–covered plate and freeze for 4 or more hours.

In a food processor, combine the banana and peanut butter and process until creamy and smooth, scraping down the blade and sides to blend.

PER SERVING	
Calories	180
Fat	8 g
Saturated fat	2 g
Cholesterol	0 mg
Sodium	75 mg
Carbohydrate	26 g
Dietary fiber	4 g
Sugars	14 g
Protein	5 g
Calcium	10 mg
Potassium	470 mg

 TIP For the family (or when the side effect has resolved), add chocolate chips before serving or try using chunky peanut butter instead of creamy.

Noodle Kugel

Every culture has its own classic comfort food. For many of Jewish descent, it's kugel, a creamy, sweet noodle casserole.

If your mouth is sore, give the noodles a few extra minutes' cooking time and bake the casserole covered the entire time to keep it very soft and tender. Otherwise, you might like to let the noodle ends get a little crunchy during baking, the way they do with baked macaroni and cheese.

If your raisins are dried out, add them to warm water for about ten minutes to plump up and soften.

Because the noodles are going to cook twice, boil them just until they soften all the way through and then run them under cold water to stop the cooking process.

To streamline cleanup, mix the ingredients in the pot the pasta cooked in instead of a mixing bowl.

6 TO 8 SERVINGS

8 ounces wide egg noodles

3 eggs

1 cup or 1 (8-ounce) container cottage cheese

1 cup or 1 (8-ounce) container sour cream

1/2 stick (4 tablespoons) butter, melted and slightly cooled

1/2 cup granulated sugar

1/2 teaspoon ground cinnamon

1/2 teaspoon vanilla extract

1/4 teaspoon salt

1/3 cup raisins

Preheat the oven to 375 degrees. Lightly coat an 8-by-8-inch (or other 1½-quart) baking pan with nonstick cooking spray.

Boil the noodles for 4 to 5 minutes, or until very al dente. Drain, rinse with cold water, drain again, and set aside.

In a food processor, pulse the eggs until combined. Add the cottage cheese, sour cream, butter, sugar, cinnamon, vanilla, and salt and process until smooth, scraping down the blade and sides to blend. Transfer to a bowl and add the noodles and raisins. Transfer the noodle mixture to the baking pan and bake for 20 to 30 minutes, or until set.

PER SERVING

Calories	460
Fat	20 g
Saturated fat	11 g
Cholesterol	180 mg
Sodium	350 mg
Carbohydrate	53 g
Dietary fiber	1 g
Sugars	24 g
Protein	14 g
Calcium	110 mg
Potassium	280 mg

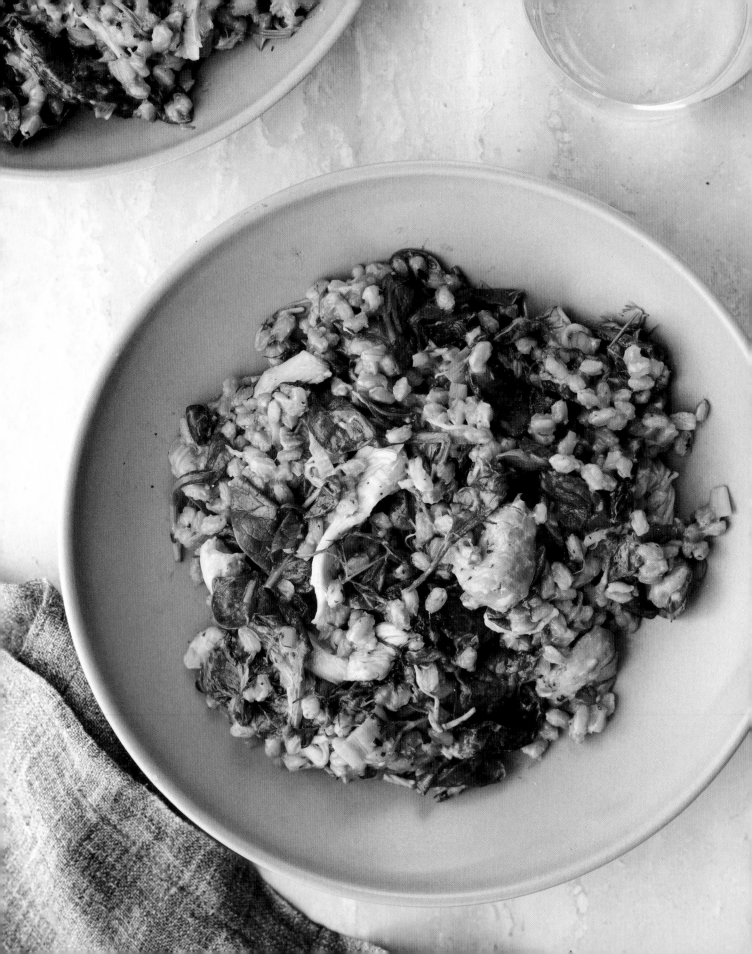

Farro "Risotto" with Chicken, Portobellos, and Spinach

Don't be misled by the name—this dish's creamy texture resembles risotto, but it is much healthier and, unlike traditional risotto, virtually hands-free to prepare. Slow cookers are ideal for longer-cooking proteins, such as chicken thighs, and for farro, a high-fiber whole grain.

Finishing the dish with greens and herbs adds freshness and a "just made" flavor often absent with slow-cooked meals. Grated Parmesan cheese provides a slightly nutty flavor, and the portobello mushrooms add an earthy note.

4 SERVINGS

1 ½ cups homemade chicken broth (page 40) or store-bought reduced-sodium broth

1 cup farro

1 pound portobello mushrooms, dark gills removed, halved and sliced

2 leeks, white and light green parts only, sliced

1 pound boneless, skinless chicken thighs, trimmed of excess fat

1 (5- to 6-ounce) package fresh baby spinach

½ cup freshly grated Parmesan cheese

¼ cup finely chopped fresh dill

Salt and freshly ground black pepper

In a slow cooker, combine the broth, farro, mushrooms, and leeks. Place the chicken on top.

Cover and cook on high for 3 to 3 ½ hours or on low for 4 to 5 hours, or until the chicken is cooked through. Stir the mixture, scraping the sides and bottom of the insert, and breaking up the chicken into smaller pieces. Add the spinach, Parmesan, and dill and stir until the spinach wilts. Season with salt and pepper.

PER SERVING	
Calories	440
Fat	11 g
Saturated fat	3.5 g
Cholesterol	110 mg
Sodium	420 mg
Carbohydrate	50 g
Dietary fiber	9 g
Sugars	4 g
Protein	34 g
Calcium	220 mg
Potassium	1200 mg

 TIP Leeks can contain a lot of dirt at their root end, so make sure to rinse them well.

C
TS
SM
WL

Rosemary–White Bean Soup

Using canned beans in this recipe allows you to skip the step of soaking beans overnight, making this soup a perfect last-minute "what's in the cupboard" meal.

Be very careful when puréeing soup in a blender or food processor. Let the soup cool slightly, don't fill the container more than two-thirds full, and secure the lid well before blending.

If the soup is too thick for your liking, add more broth or water.

6 SERVINGS

1 tablespoon canola oil

1 onion, chopped

1 carrot, chopped

1 celery stalk, chopped

2 garlic cloves, finely chopped

4 cups homemade chicken or vegetable broth (pages 40 or 74) or store-bought reduced-sodium broth

3 (15-ounce) cans navy or Great Northern beans, rinsed and drained

1 (4-inch) sprig fresh rosemary

Salt and freshly ground black pepper

In a stockpot over medium-high heat, add the oil. Sauté the onion, carrot, and celery for 5 to 7 minutes, or until softened. Add the garlic and sauté for 1 to 2 minutes. Add the broth and beans and stir to combine. Bring to a boil. Reduce the heat, add the rosemary, and simmer for 20 to 25 minutes, stirring occasionally. Cool slightly and remove the rosemary sprig.

Transfer to a blender or food processor and purée (you may need to do this step in two or more batches). Season with salt and pepper.

PER SERVING

Calories	210
Fat	3.5 g
Saturated fat	0.5 g
Cholesterol	4 mg
Sodium	600 mg
Carbohydrate	34 g
Dietary fiber	13 g
Sugars	2 g
Protein	12 g
Calcium	100 mg
Potassium	560 mg

TIP This recipe may not be suitable if you are experiencing gas or bloating.

Mini Chicken Pot Pies

These miniature pies are sized for single servings. Keep extra cooked pies in the fridge to heat up for individual meals or freeze for later use. You will need four ramekins or oven-safe teacups for this recipe—they should hold at least one cup.

4 SERVINGS

1 pound boneless, skinless chicken breasts, halved

1 cup milk

2 tablespoons butter

1 small (or ½ large) onion, finely chopped

2 tablespoons all-purpose flour

1 cup homemade chicken broth (page 40) or store-bought reduced-sodium broth

1 cup frozen peas and carrots

Salt and freshly ground black pepper

1 refrigerated roll-out pie crust

1 egg combined with 1 tablespoon water, optional

Preheat the oven to 350 degrees.

In a baking pan, place the chicken in a single layer and add milk. Bake for 25 to 30 minutes, or until chicken is just cooked through. Remove the chicken and set aside to cool briefly, reserving the milk. Cut chicken into bite-sized pieces.

Increase the oven temperature to 425 degrees.

Meanwhile, in a large saucepan over medium heat, melt the butter. Sauté the onion for 3 to 5 minutes, or until softened. Add the flour and cook until fully incorporated, stirring constantly. Gradually add the broth and cook until thickened, stirring constantly. Add the reserved milk and cook until thickened. Add the peas and carrots and the chicken. Season with salt and pepper.

Divide chicken mixture evenly between four (1-cup) ramekins or oven-safe teacups. Roll out the crust and cut four circles; the circles should be big enough to overlap the edges of the ramekins by about 1 inch on all sides, but they need not be perfect circles. Top each ramekin with crust, pressing to seal the sides.

Brush the tops of the pies with the egg mixture, if desired. Cut a slit in the top of each crust. Place the ramekins on a baking sheet.

Bake for 12 to 18 minutes, or until the tops are golden. Let cool for 5 to 10 minutes before serving.

PER SERVING	
Calories	420
Fat	21 g
Saturated fat	9 g
Cholesterol	90 mg
Sodium	480 mg
Carbohydrate	28 g
Dietary fiber	2 g
Sugars	7 g
Protein	30 g
Calcium	110 mg
Potassium	420 mg

Simple Herb Risotto

There are few things as comforting as a bowl of creamy risotto. The rice expands with the liquid to soften and take on a porridge-like consistency.

Although this risotto tastes rich, it actually contains almost no fat, unlike restaurant versions that can be loaded with butter and heavy cream. The herbs add vibrancy. If you are experiencing diarrhea, add one-quarter cup herbs and have family members add more to their individual portions.

While it is not essential to warm the broth first, it helps maintain an even cooking temperature. If you prefer not to cook with wine, replace it with additional broth.

4 SERVINGS

4 cups homemade chicken or vegetable broth (pages 40 or 74) or store-bought reduced-sodium broth

1 tablespoon olive oil

2 shallots or ½ onion, finely chopped

1 cup Arborio, Carnaroli, or "risotto" rice

½ cup dry white wine

1 cup (packed) finely chopped fresh herbs (such as Italian parsley, dill, thyme, cilantro, and/or basil)

Salt and freshly ground black pepper

In a saucepan, bring the broth to a simmer. Cover and keep warm over low heat. (You can also microwave the broth.)

In a large stockpot over medium heat, add the oil. Sauté the shallots for 3 to 5 minutes. Add the rice and sauté for 1 minute. Increase the heat to medium-high, add the wine, and stir constantly until it is almost completely absorbed. Begin slowly adding the broth, ½ cup at a time, stirring frequently. Wait until the liquid is almost completely absorbed before adding more, 2 to 4 minutes. Continue to add broth for 20 to 30 minutes, or until the rice is soft and the risotto has a creamy texture, stirring frequently. You may not need to use all of the broth.

Add the herbs and stir to combine. Season with salt and pepper. Serve immediately.

PER SERVING

Calories	220
Fat	4.5 g
Saturated fat	0.5 g
Cholesterol	6 mg
Sodium	500 mg
Carbohydrate	36 g
Dietary fiber	2 g
Sugars	0.5 g
Protein	5 g
Calcium	20 mg
Potassium	110 mg

 TIP For the family (or when side effect has resolved), add Parmesan cheese. For a heartier meal with protein, top with cooked chicken, shrimp, or fish.

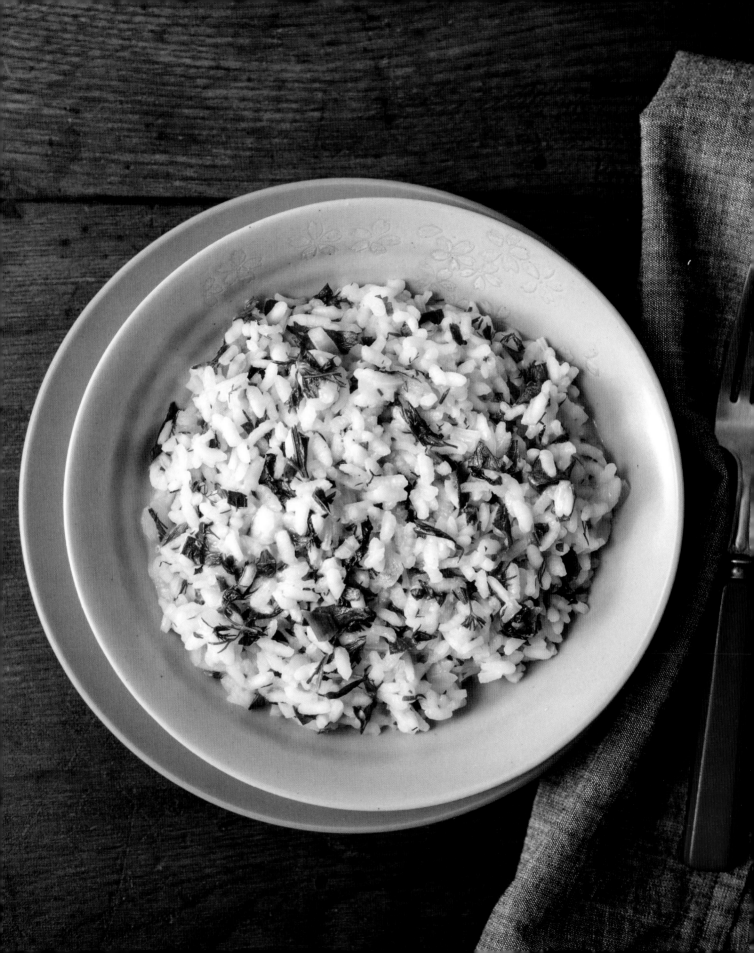

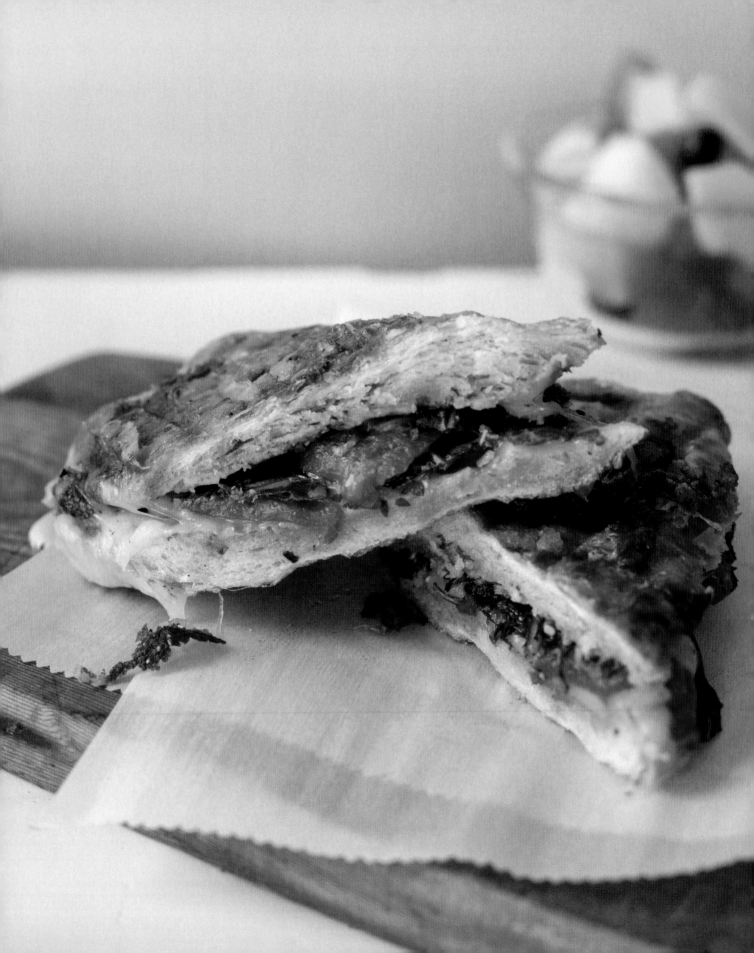

WL UNINTENTIONAL WEIGHT LOSS

Acai-Banana-Raspberry Smoothie Bowl

Fortified Milk

Banana-Yogurt Quick Bread

Creamy Mac and Cheese with Broccoli

Almond-Date Energy Orbs

Spinach-Artichoke Dip Quesadillas

Turkey-Quinoa Not-Too-Sloppy Joes

Beef and Spinach Lasagna with Parmesan Sauce

Good Old-Fashioned Cheese Balls

Mozzarella, Pesto, and Roasted Red Pepper Panini

Fruity Chicken Salad

Spaghetti with Silky Avocado-Basil Sauce

Breakfast "Banana Split"

Double-Cheese Polenta "Plank" Pizzas

Peanut Noodles

Chocolate Chip-Raisin Granola Bars

Cheesy French Toast

Peanut Butter–Banana–Chocolate Panini

Grain Bowl with Spinach, Pickled Carrots, and Fried Egg

UNINTENTIONAL WEIGHT LOSS REFERS TO WEIGHT LOSS THAT OCCURS WITHOUT DIETING. This can happen for a number of reasons: some types of cancer and cancer treatment may increase your overall nutritional needs, you might not feel hungry or have any desire to eat, or you are experiencing challenging side effects from treatment. Maintaining your weight can be difficult in the face of any of these issues. Even if you are overweight, weight loss during cancer treatment can increase fatigue, decrease your strength, affect your immune system, lengthen recovery times, and decrease your quality of life. Unintentional weight loss during this time usually reflects a loss of muscle rather than fat, which can place you at higher risk for malnutrition and can affect your ability to carry out normal daily activities.

If you are trying to prevent weight loss, maintain your weight, or gain weight, it is important to talk with your health care team to get help. You may need to find ways to increase both calories and protein in your diet. This often means choosing calorie- and protein-rich foods or adjusting recipes by adding extra protein or higher-calorie alternatives. For example, one of the first recipes in this chapter is for Fortified Milk, which can be used in recipes in place of regular milk to add calories and protein. You may also need to eat more frequently: if you can eat more often throughout the day, even if it's a small amount at a time, it will be easier to prevent weight loss.

Here are some ideas to help you increase the amount of calories and protein in your diet:

- Eat five to six small meals or snacks a day, or try to eat a little something every two to three hours.

- Try to choose nutritious snacks that are high in calories and/or protein, such as trail mix, nuts, dried fruit, granola, hard-boiled eggs, peanut butter or other nut butters, hummus, cottage cheese, yogurt, cheese, and canned tuna or chicken.

- Try smoothies, milk shakes, or nutritional supplements or bars to add more calories and protein to your diet.

- If you get full quickly, try sipping your liquids between meals so that you are not so full at meal times.

- Eat your favorite foods any time of the day.

- Adding higher-calorie foods such as sour cream, cream cheese, whipped cream, butter, and gravy may be helpful in the short term to avoid further weight loss. Many favorite recipes can be easily altered to increase the amount of calories and protein they contain.

- Try eating when you are the hungriest—for many people, this is in the morning.

- Do not limit yourself to traditional meals when it comes to what and when you eat. It is perfectly okay to have breakfast food for lunch or supper for breakfast.

- Ask friends and family for help with shopping and making meals and snacks to help keep you stocked with things to eat and drink.

If you are trying to gain weight or prevent weight loss, the goal should simply be to eat as many healthful calories and protein-rich foods as possible, as well as to enjoy eating as much as you can. It is important to note that weight fluctuations are typical. You may lose weight and have a relatively poor appetite the week after chemotherapy, but gain most or all of it back before your next treatment.

Be sure to tell your health care team if you have changes in your weight. If your weight loss is accompanied by a poor appetite, your doctor may prescribe medicine to help stimulate your appetite and improve your food and beverage intake.

CONTACT YOUR DOCTOR IN THESE SITUATIONS:

- You have weight loss of three or more pounds in one week.

- You have ongoing weight loss without trying.

For more information about managing unintentional weight loss, visit the American Cancer Society website at cancer.org or call 800-227-2345.

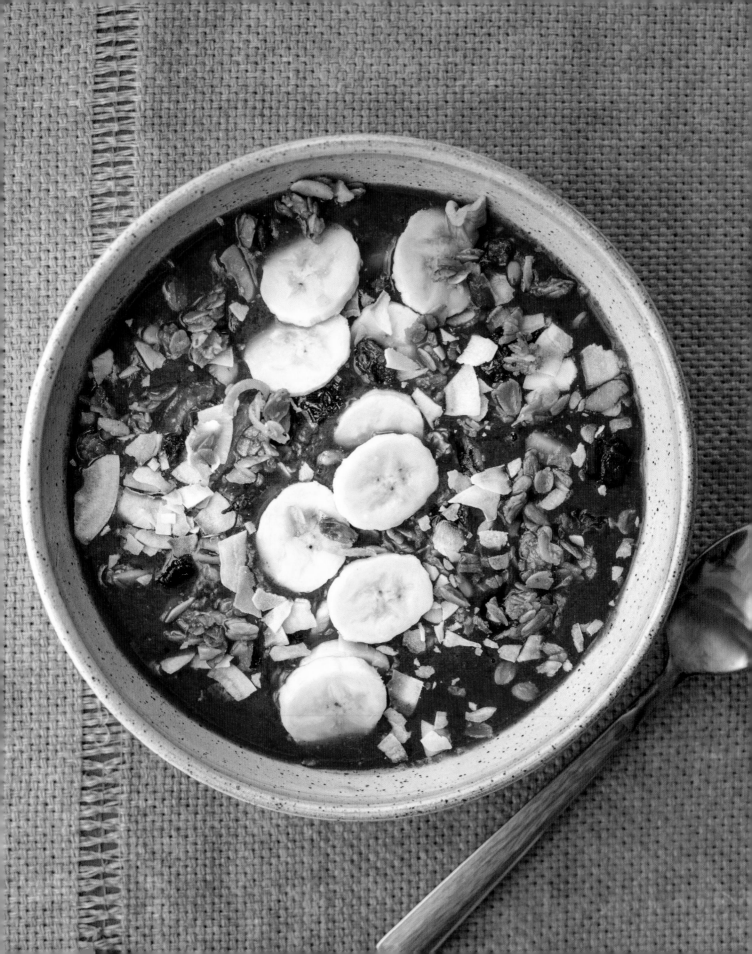

Acai-Banana-Raspberry Smoothie Bowl

An acai (ah-sigh-e) bowl is basically a smoothie so thick it's served in a bowl and eaten with a spoon. Acai, a purple, bitter, berrylike fruit, is packed with antioxidants and omega-3 fatty acids, in addition to fiber and other nutrients.

A staple in Brazil that's now making its way north, acai purée is sold in packets in the frozen fruit section of many supermarkets. It's typically puréed with other ingredients to sweeten it and, reminiscent of the frozen yogurt craze, the mixture acts as a base for toppings galore. Popular add-ons include granola, fresh or dried fruit, and coconut, to add flavor and texture—and, for those in need, extra calories.

If you have trouble finding acai, you can make any smoothie a smoothie bowl by reducing the amount of liquid when blending and serving it with toppings.

For best results, use a high-speed blender such as a Vitamix. For a thicker puree, put the banana in the freezer for an hour or two before blending.

2 SERVINGS

1 (110g/3.53-ounce) acai purée pouch, broken up in pieces

1/2 cup 100 percent apple or white grape juice

1 banana, sliced

1 cup frozen raspberries or cherries

Fresh berries, sliced bananas, granola, dried fruit, toasted coconut, chopped nuts, optional

Run the acai pouch under warm water until it can be broken up into pieces. In a blender, combine the apple juice, banana, acai, and raspberries and blend for 30 to 60 seconds, or until smooth. Pour into individual bowls and add toppings, if desired.

PER SERVING

Calories	170
Fat	3.5 g
Saturated fat	1 g
Cholesterol	0 mg
Sodium	10 mg
Carbohydrate	35 g
Dietary fiber	4 g
Sugars	25 g
Protein	3 g
Calcium	50 mg
Potassium	500 mg

Fortified Milk

Fortifying milk with nonfat instant dry milk adds protein and calories to your diet. Drink the milk by itself, add to a milk shake, or use in place of regular milk when making shakes, macaroni and cheese, puddings, and mashed potatoes.

If the taste is too strong, dilute with liquid milk until palatable, or start with one-half cup of dry milk and gradually work up to one cup.

4 SERVINGS

1 quart low-fat milk   1 cup nonfat dry milk

In a container, blend low-fat milk and dry milk until dissolved. Cover and refrigerate for at least 6 hours.

PER SERVING

Calories	160
Fat	2.5 g
Saturated fat	1.5 g
Cholesterol	15 mg
Sodium	200 mg
Carbohydrate	21 g
Dietary fiber	0 g
Sugars	21 g
Protein	14 g
Calcium	500 mg
Potassium	660 mg

Banana-Yogurt Quick Bread

Using whole wheat and buckwheat flours instead of refined white flour gives this banana bread an earthier flavor. Despite the name, buckwheat is actually not in the wheat family. It's a grain-like seed in the rhubarb family and is an excellent source of fiber, protein, and other nutrients.

After cooling, top the slices with peanut or almond butter for added protein, healthy fat, and calories.

When you are preparing any batter, make sure to periodically scrape the sides and bottom of the mixing bowl to incorporate it for more uniform blending.

10 SERVINGS

1 cup whole wheat flour

1/2 cup buckwheat flour

2 teaspoons ground cinnamon

1 teaspoon baking soda

1/2 teaspoon baking powder

1/2 teaspoon salt

1/2 cup olive oil

3/4 cup light brown sugar

2 eggs

1/2 cup plain Greek yogurt

4 ripe bananas

Preheat the oven to 350 degrees. Coat a 9-by-5-by-3-inch loaf pan with nonstick cooking spray. Line the bottom of the pan with parchment paper.

In a bowl, combine the whole wheat flour, buckwheat flour, cinnamon, baking soda, baking powder, and salt.

In a bowl, using an electric mixer, blend the oil and brown sugar. Add the eggs one at a time. Add the yogurt and beat until combined. Add the banana and beat until blended but still chunky. Add the dry ingredients and beat on low until just combined, scraping down the beater(s) and sides to blend. Do not overmix.

Scrape the batter into the pan and smooth the top with a spatula.

Bake for 50 to 60 minutes, or until the top is firm and a toothpick inserted in the center comes out clean. Cool in the pan on a rack for 10 to 15 minutes. Use a knife or spatula to loosen the sides of the loaf from the pan before removing. Cool completely on the rack before slicing.

PER SERVING	
Calories	270
Fat	13 g
Saturated fat	2 g
Cholesterol	40 mg
Sodium	280 mg
Carbohydrate	36 g
Dietary fiber	4 g
Sugars	17 g
Protein	5 g
Calcium	60 mg
Potassium	310 mg

 TIP Lining the bottom of the baking pan with parchment paper makes removing the quick bread easier.

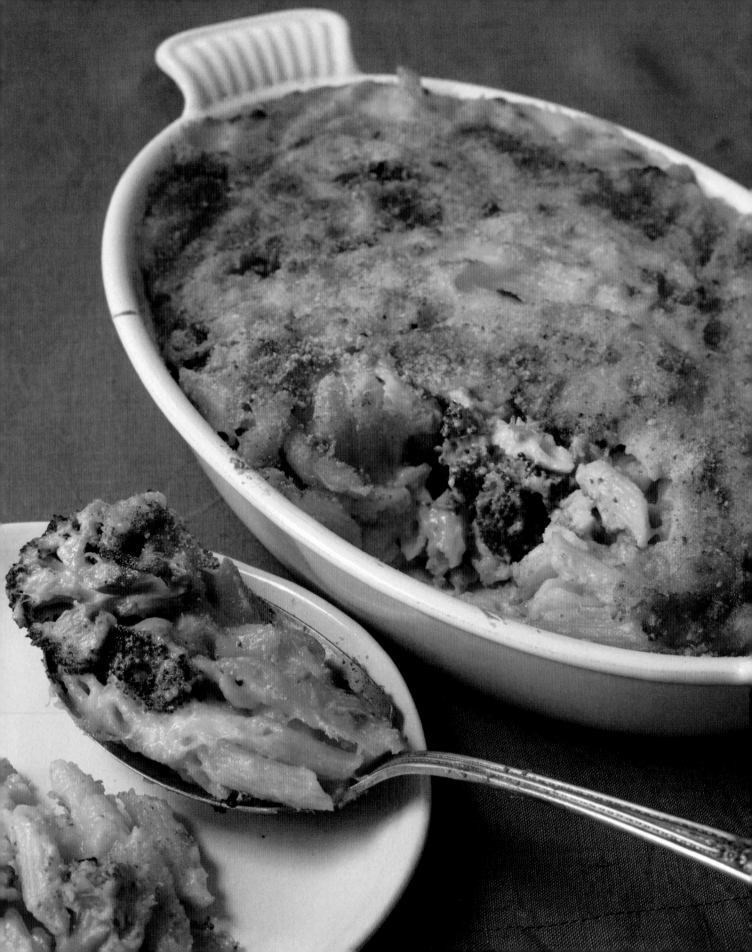

Creamy Mac and Cheese with Broccoli

Who doesn't crave mac and cheese when we aren't feeling our best and want something comforting? This casserole delivers that homey, cheesy creaminess in every bite. The addition of chopped broccoli adds texture and vitamins and makes it a complete meal.

Don't be concerned if the pasta is still a little firm after boiling. It will finish softening during baking.

6 SERVINGS

8 ounces shaped pasta, such as elbows, small shells, or mini penne

3 cups chopped broccoli

2 tablespoons butter

1 small onion, finely chopped

2 tablespoons all-purpose flour

½ teaspoon dry mustard

1 ½ cups whole milk

3 cups shredded sharp Cheddar cheese

1 cup grated Parmesan cheese, divided use

Salt and freshly ground black pepper

1 tablespoon bread crumbs

Preheat the oven to 350 degrees. Lightly coat an 8-by-8-inch or other 1 ½- to 2-quart baking pan with nonstick cooking spray.

Cook the pasta until very al dente, about 4 minutes. Add the broccoli and cook for 1 minute. Drain, rinse with cold water, drain again, and set aside.

Meanwhile, in a saucepan over medium-low heat, melt the butter. Add the onion and sauté for 3 to 5 minutes, or until softened. Add the flour and mustard and whisk constantly for 1 minute to incorporate. When the mixture turns golden, gradually add the milk and bring to a boil, whisking constantly. Reduce the heat and simmer for 2 to 3 minutes or until thickened and smooth, whisking frequently. Add the Cheddar and stir to combine. Reserve 1 tablespoon of the Parmesan and add the rest to the sauce. Stir until combined.

If room allows, add the reserved pasta and broccoli to the saucepan and stir to combine (if the pan isn't big enough, you can mix it all in a bowl). Season with salt and pepper.

Transfer to the baking pan and sprinkle with the bread crumbs and the reserved 1 tablespoon Parmesan.

Cover with foil and bake for 20 minutes. Uncover and bake for 5 minutes.

PER SERVING	
Calories	530
Fat	29 g
Saturated fat	17 g
Cholesterol	85 mg
Sodium	600 mg
Carbohydrate	41 g
Dietary fiber	3 g
Sugars	6 g
Protein	28 g
Calcium	650 mg
Potassium	360 mg

 TIP If broccoli is too hard on your stomach, omit it, or substitute another favorite vegetable or protein, such as cooked squash, green peas, tuna, or beans.

Almond-Date Energy Orbs

Plump dried Medjool dates, often found in the refrigerated section of the supermarket, are so sweet you would swear you were eating candy. Not only are they delicious to snack on by themselves, their creamy, caramel-like interior makes them perfect for mixing into shakes or snacks, like these no-cook confections. Oats and almond butter add protein and fiber.

Squeezing the mixture (instead of rolling it) helps the balls stay together. Store extras in an airtight container in the fridge for snacking throughout the day.

12 SERVINGS

½ cup old-fashioned rolled oats

½ cup almond butter

4 Medjool dates, pitted

1 to 2 tablespoons pure maple syrup

¼ cup unsweetened coconut

2 tablespoons ground flaxseeds

½ teaspoon ground cinnamon

In a food processor, pulse the oats several times until they resemble large crumbs. Add the almond butter, dates, and 1 tablespoon of the maple syrup and pulse until the dates are fully chopped and everything is combined. Taste and add maple syrup, if desired. Add the coconut, flaxseeds, and cinnamon and process until combined, scraping down the blade and sides to blend. Squeeze into 1-inch balls.

PER SERVING

Calories	130
Fat	8 g
Saturated fat	1.5 g
Cholesterol	0 mg
Sodium	0 mg
Carbohydrate	13 g
Dietary fiber	4 g
Sugars	7 g
Protein	3 g
Calcium	50 mg
Potassium	170 mg

Spinach–Artichoke Dip Quesadillas

Here's a twist on everyone's favorite party dip. While it's delicious on its own or eaten with crudité or crackers, sandwiching it between two tortillas and heating it makes it an easy-to-eat snack or small meal.

Dry the artichokes and spinach well to keep the mixture from getting too waterlogged.

6 SERVINGS

1 cup canned artichoke hearts in water, drained, quartered, and patted dry

4 ounces cream cheese, room temperature

¼ cup freshly grated Parmesan cheese

1 tablespoon fresh lemon juice

Pinch ground nutmeg

8 ounces frozen chopped spinach, defrosted and squeezed dry

2 cups shredded mozzarella cheese

Salt and freshly ground black pepper

12 (5- to 6-inch) whole wheat or corn tortillas

Preheat the oven to 300 degrees.

In a food processor, pulse the artichoke hearts until coarsely chopped. Add the cream cheese, Parmesan, lemon juice, and nutmeg and pulse until combined. Add the spinach and mozzarella cheese and pulse until incorporated, scraping down the blade and sides to blend. Season with salt and pepper.

Divide the mixture onto six tortillas. Top with the remaining tortillas.

Lightly coat a nonstick skillet with nonstick cooking spray and place over medium heat. Add the quesadillas one at a time and cook for 3 to 5 minutes per side, or until crisp on the outside and warm throughout. Transfer to a baking sheet to keep warm in the oven while cooking the remaining quesadillas.

PER SERVING	
Calories	370
Fat	19 g
Saturated fat	11 g
Cholesterol	45 mg
Sodium	730 mg
Carbohydrate	32 g
Dietary fiber	8 g
Sugars	3 g
Protein	19 g
Calcium	530 mg
Potassium	370 mg

Turkey-Quinoa Not-Too-Sloppy Joes

This sloppy joe filling is a little thicker than most so it stays nicely tucked in the bun. The unexpected addition of quinoa adds texture in addition to beneficial fiber, protein, and other nutrients.

Prepare this when you have leftover quinoa on hand, or make the quinoa fresh. Start it when you begin the recipe and it will be ready when you need it. If cooking quinoa for this recipe, make extra to serve with Chicken Tagine with Carrots, Prunes, and Chickpeas (page 104) or to use in the Grain Bowl with Spinach, Pickled Carrots, and Fried Egg (page 216).

6 SERVINGS

1 tablespoon olive oil

1 onion, finely chopped

1 red or green bell pepper, seeded and chopped

2 garlic cloves, minced

2 teaspoons ground chili powder

1½ teaspoons ground cumin

¼ teaspoon ground cinnamon

1 pound ground turkey

2 (8-ounce) cans tomato sauce

3 tablespoons tomato paste

1 cup cooked quinoa

Salt and freshly ground black pepper

4 hamburger buns, lightly toasted

In a large skillet over medium-high heat, add the oil. Sauté the onion and bell pepper for 5 to 7 minutes, or until softened. Add the garlic, chili powder, cumin, and cinnamon and sauté for 1 to 2 minutes, or until the spices are fragrant. Add the turkey and sauté for 5 to 8 minutes, or until cooked through, breaking it up into small pieces with a spatula. Add the tomato sauce and tomato paste and bring to a boil, stirring to combine. Reduce the heat and simmer for 10 minutes, or until the sauce thickens, stirring occasionally. Add the quinoa and season with salt and pepper. Serve on toasted buns.

PER SERVING

Calories	300
Fat	10 g
Saturated fat	2 g
Cholesterol	50 mg
Sodium	620 mg
Carbohydrate	31 g
Dietary fiber	4 g
Sugars	8 g
Protein	21 g
Calcium	100 mg
Potassium	670 mg

TIP For added calories, top sandwiches with grated Cheddar cheese or melt some on the bun before serving.

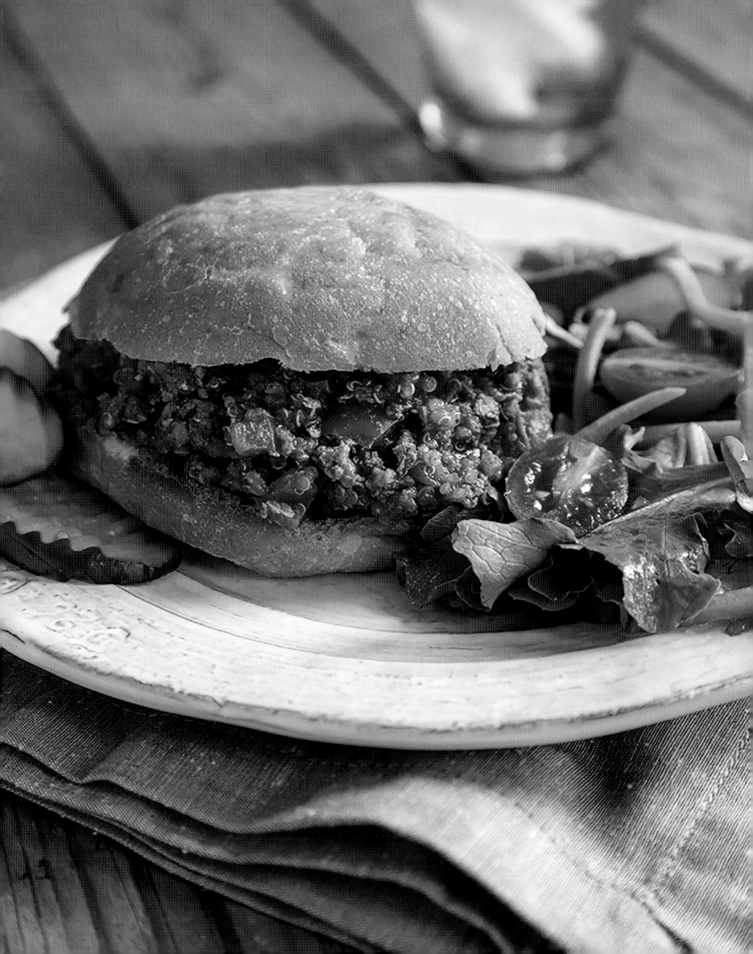

Beef and Spinach Lasagna with Parmesan Sauce

This creamy pasta casserole uses a béchamel sauce instead of mozzarella for a rich, comforting, and satisfying meal that's lighter than a typical lasagna.

8 SERVINGS

1 tablespoon olive oil

1 onion, finely chopped

2 garlic cloves, minced

1 pound lean ground beef

1 (5- to 6-ounce) package fresh baby spinach

1 (28-ounce) can crushed tomatoes

Salt and freshly ground black pepper

4 tablespoons butter

¼ cup all-purpose flour

3 cups milk

1 ½ cups freshly grated Parmesan cheese, divided use

12 no-boil lasagna noodles

Place one oven rack in the top setting and the other in the middle slot. Preheat the oven to 350 degrees. Lightly coat a 9-by-13-inch (or other 2-quart) baking pan with nonstick cooking spray.

In a large skillet over medium-high heat, add the oil. Sauté the onion for 3 to 5 minutes, or until softened. Add the garlic and sauté for 1 minute. Add the ground beef and sauté for 5 to 8 minutes, or until cooked through, using a spatula to break it up into small pieces. Add the spinach, a bit at a time, and sauté for 1 to 2 minutes, or until wilted. Add the tomatoes and bring to a boil, stirring to combine. Reduce the heat and simmer for 10 minutes, or until thickened, stirring occasionally. Season with salt and pepper.

Meanwhile, in a saucepan over medium-low heat, melt the butter. Add the flour and whisk constantly for 1 minute to incorporate. When the mixture turns golden, gradually add the milk and bring to a boil, whisking constantly. Reduce the heat and simmer for 2 to 3 minutes, or until thickened and smooth, whisking frequently. Add 1 cup of the Parmesan and whisk to combine. Season with salt and pepper.

Arrange one layer of lasagna noodles in the baking pan. Top with half of the tomato mixture and one-third of the white sauce. Repeat. Top with a layer of noodles and the remaining white sauce. Sprinkle with the remaining ½ cup of Parmesan. Cover with foil and bake for 30 minutes, or until heated through. Remove the foil and change to the broil setting. Transfer the baking pan to the top shelf and broil for 30 to 60 seconds, rotating once, until bubbly and golden brown in spots, watching to prevent burning.

PER SERVING	
Calories	420
Fat	20 g
Saturated fat	10 g
Cholesterol	90 mg
Sodium	460 mg
Carbohydrate	36 g
Dietary fiber	3 g
Sugars	11 g
Protein	25 g
Calcium	340 mg
Potassium	790 mg

Good Old-Fashioned Cheese Balls

Some snacks never go out of style, and these retro cheese balls are a great example. You can make smaller portions to nibble on or roll the cheese mixture into one larger ball and slice it to serve with crackers. If making one large ball, scrape the mixture onto plastic wrap and form into a ball, sealing well. Refrigerate for two or more hours, or until firm. Right before serving, remove the plastic wrap and roll the ball(s) in the nuts, pressing well to adhere.

This cheese mixture is especially good if you are having mouth issues: omit the nuts and cut back on, or eliminate, the seasonings. Alternatively, if you prefer a sharper-flavored spread, increase the amounts of onion powder and garlic powder, to taste.

12 SERVINGS

4 ounces cream cheese, softened

1/2 cup (2 ounces) shredded sharp Cheddar cheese

1/2 cup (2 ounces) freshly grated Parmesan cheese

1/2 cup (2 ounces) crumbled goat cheese

1/2 teaspoon garlic powder

1/4 teaspoon onion powder

1/3 cup finely chopped toasted pistachios, pecans, or walnuts, optional

In a bowl, using an electric mixer, blend the cream cheese, Cheddar, Parmesan, goat cheese, garlic powder, and onion powder for 1 minute, or until smooth, scraping down the beater(s) and sides to blend. Roll the mixture into golf ball-sized portions. Refrigerate for 1 or more hours, or until firm. Roll in the pistachios, if desired, pressing to coat.

PER SERVING (ONE BALL)	
Calories	80
Fat	7 g
Saturated fat	4 g
Cholesterol	20 mg
Sodium	115 mg
Carbohydrate	1 g
Dietary fiber	0 g
Sugars	0 g
Protein	4 g
Calcium	90 mg
Potassium	20 mg

TIP If experiencing neutropenia, substitute additional cream cheese for the goat cheese and use regular Cheddar instead of sharp Cheddar.

Mozzarella, Pesto, and Roasted Red Pepper Panini

Let's face it: paninis just taste good. Maybe it's the warm and gooey insides, or maybe the grill marks and the bits of crusty Parmesan flecking the top make this sandwich seem special.

This salute to Italy, with its red, green, and white layers, has robust flavor in addition to providing necessary calories when you're rebuilding during and after treatment. If you aren't a fan of roasted red peppers, substitute sun-dried tomatoes.

If you don't have a panini maker, don't worry. This can easily be made on the stovetop. If using a skillet, sprinkle the Parmesan on the pesto before layering the cheese. Cook until the bottom is golden brown, pressing the top firmly with a spatula to condense the sandwich. Carefully turn the sandwich and cook until the bottom is golden brown.

2 TO 3 SERVINGS

2 tablespoons pesto

2 (4- to 6-inch) crusty rolls or a baguette, cut in half lengthwise

4 ounces mozzarella cheese, sliced or grated

1 roasted red bell pepper, cut into strips

1 cup arugula

1 tablespoon freshly grated Parmesan cheese

Preheat the panini press.

Spread the pesto on the top and bottom of the cut side of the rolls. On the bottom slices, divide the mozzarella and top with the roasted red pepper and arugula. Cover with the top of the roll.

Place in the panini press, close to flatten, and cook for 1 to 2 minutes. Once the rolls are flattened, lift the press and sprinkle the Parmesan on the top of the rolls. Press down and cook for 3 to 5 minutes, or until both sides are golden brown and the cheese has melted.

PER SERVING	
Calories	400
Fat	15 g
Saturated fat	7 g
Cholesterol	40 mg
Sodium	940 mg
Carbohydrate	43 g
Dietary fiber	3 g
Sugars	4 g
Protein	24 g
Calcium	520 mg
Potassium	220 mg

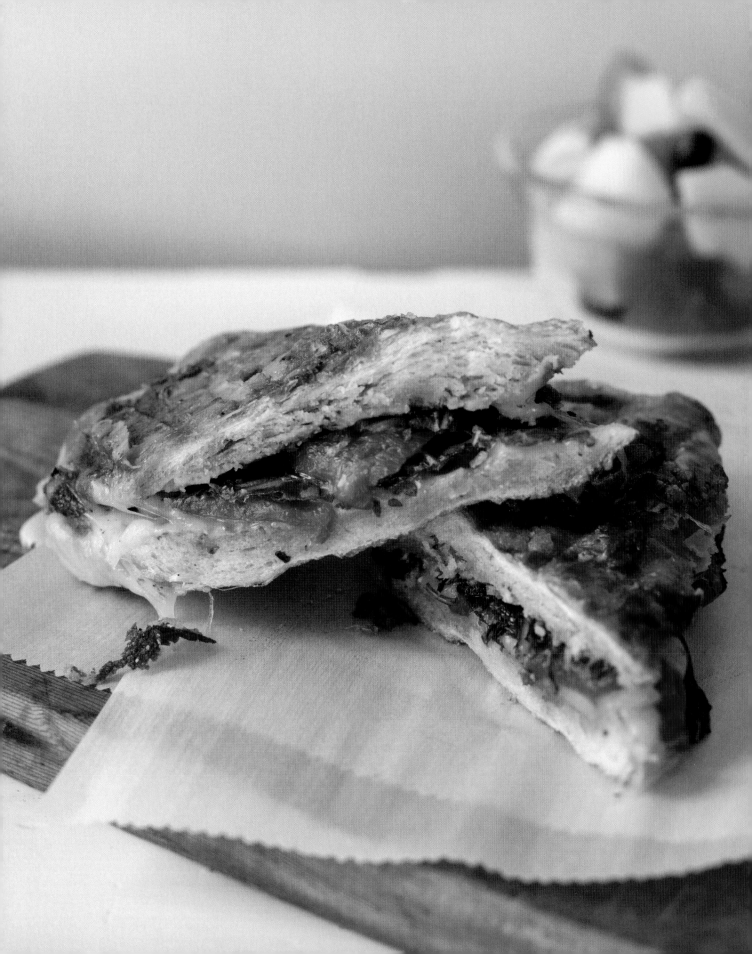

Fruity Chicken Salad

Each bite of this salad provides a burst of flavor and texture from the mixture of chicken, dried sweetened cranberries, crunchy apples, and toasted almonds.

If you want to avoid mayonnaise, substitute a vinaigrette or Italian dressing. If you want something a little sweeter, substitute vanilla yogurt.

While not essential, adding fresh herbs gives the salad vibrancy. If you have some in your fridge or garden, snip a few leaves.

4 SERVINGS

2 cups (about 8 ounces) chopped cooked chicken

2 scallions, thinly sliced

1 apple, chopped

1 celery stalk, finely chopped

¼ cup dried sweetened cranberries

2 to 3 tablespoons regular or reduced-fat mayonnaise

2 tablespoons chopped fresh basil or Italian parsley or 1 tablespoon chopped fresh tarragon, optional

Salt and freshly ground black pepper

¼ cup slivered almonds, toasted

In a bowl, combine the chicken, scallions, apple, celery, cranberries, and 2 tablespoons of the mayonnaise. Add the herbs, if desired, and stir gently to incorporate. Add more mayonnaise if necessary. Season with salt and pepper. Add the toasted almonds just before serving. If you're not eating all of the salad at once, add the nuts to individual servings right before eating to keep them crunchy.

PER SERVING

Calories	250
Fat	13 g
Saturated fat	2 g
Cholesterol	50 mg
Sodium	100 mg
Carbohydrate	14 g
Dietary fiber	3 g
Sugars	10 g
Protein	18 g
Calcium	40 mg
Potassium	290 mg

TIP Toasting nuts brings out their flavor and adds crunch. Bake at 350 degrees for about 5 minutes, or toast in a skillet until golden. Cool before using.

Spaghetti with Silky Avocado-Basil Sauce

Don't believe it's not easy being green! This dish is not only a snap to make, it's delicious and filled with good-for-you fats from creamy, ripe avocados. To mellow the flavor of the garlic, blanch it in the boiling water for one minute, removing it before adding the pasta. If you set the water up to boil before you begin the recipe, the pasta will finish cooking in the time that it takes to make the sauce. The heat of the pasta warms the sauce so there's only one pot to clean.

If tomatoes are in season, top the finished dish with a few quartered cherry tomatoes or, for added calories, toasted pine nuts and a generous drizzle of olive oil. For added protein, top with cooked chicken or shrimp.

4 SERVINGS

2 garlic cloves

12 ounces spaghetti

½ cup fresh basil leaves

2 ripe avocados, halved and pitted

2 tablespoons fresh lemon juice

1 tablespoon extra-virgin olive oil

Salt and freshly ground black pepper

Fill a stockpot two-thirds full of water and bring to a boil. Add the garlic and cook for 1 minute. Remove and set aside.

In the same pot, prepare the spaghetti according to the package directions for al dente (just firm). Reserve ¼ cup of the pasta water before draining. Set aside.

Meanwhile, in a food processor, pulse the blanched garlic and basil until finely chopped. Scrape in the avocado flesh, lemon juice, and olive oil and process until smooth, scraping down the blade and sides to blend. Season with salt and pepper.

In a bowl, combine the reserved pasta and the sauce and stir to combine. If too dry, add reserved pasta water 1 tablespoon at a time, stirring to combine.

PER SERVING	
Calories	470
Fat	16 g
Saturated fat	2 g
Cholesterol	0 mg
Sodium	15 mg
Carbohydrate	72 g
Dietary fiber	8 g
Sugars	3 g
Protein	13 g
Calcium	40 mg
Potassium	590 mg

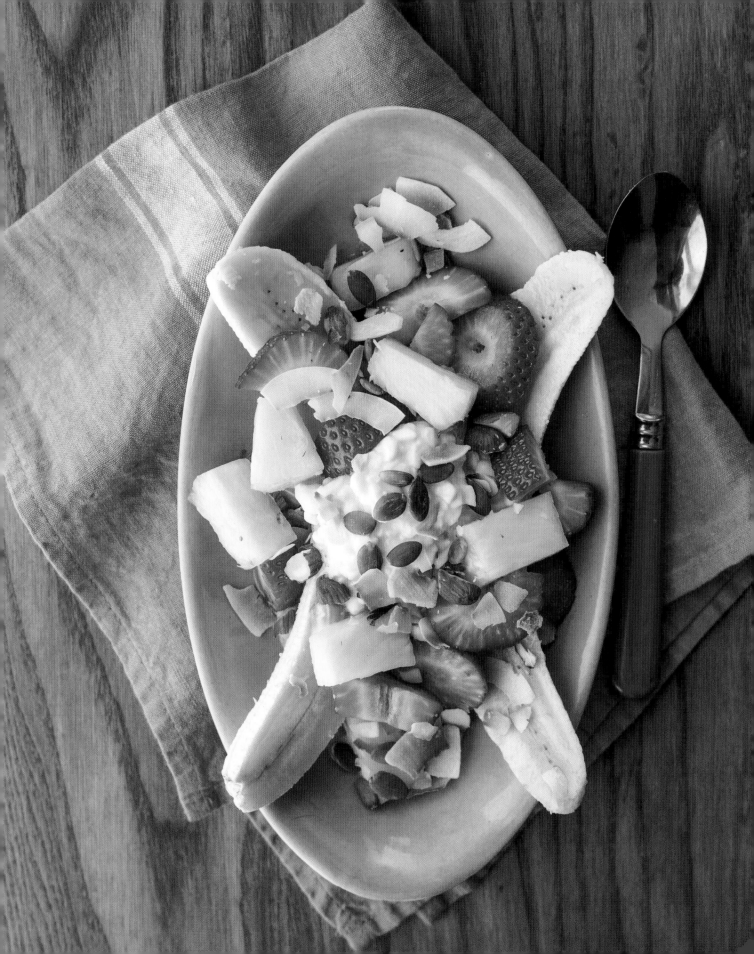

Breakfast "Banana Split"

If your appetite isn't what it once was, a little whimsy can make mealtime a little easier to face. This riff on the popular ice cream parlor dessert is a good choice for any time of day.

Calcium- and protein-rich cottage cheese, Greek yogurt, or a combination of the two subs for ice cream. Instead of topping the mixture with sugary syrups, an assortment of fresh fruit, nuts, seeds, and toasted coconut adds crunch and natural sweetness.

The combinations of flavors and textures make this small meal go a long way.

1 SERVING

½ cup cottage cheese, plain Greek yogurt, or a combination

1 tablespoon honey

½ ripe banana, cut in half lengthwise

3 strawberries, sliced

1 (1-inch) "ring" fresh pineapple, cut into ½-inch pieces

4 roasted unsalted almonds, chopped

1 teaspoon toasted unsweetened coconut

1 teaspoon roasted unsalted pepitas (pumpkin seeds) or sunflower seeds, optional

In a shallow bowl, mound a scoop of cottage cheese and drizzle with honey. Place the banana halves on two sides and top with strawberries and pineapple. Sprinkle with almonds, coconut, and pepitas, if desired.

PER SERVING

Calories	340
Fat	9 g
Saturated fat	3 g
Cholesterol	20 mg
Sodium	400 mg
Carbohydrate	54 g
Dietary fiber	5 g
Sugars	41 g
Protein	15 g
Calcium	130 mg
Potassium	580 mg

Double-Cheese Polenta "Plank" Pizzas

If you are having gluten sensitivity or are looking for a twist on a classic dish, try these "mini pizzas" that use sliced store-bought polenta as a crust instead of a traditional dough made with flour.

Broil the "planks" first for crispness and a little charred flavor before topping them with sauce and cheese. Use your favorite jarred marinara sauce or make your own with the recipe below. The whole meal takes less than thirty minutes to prepare!

4 SERVINGS

1 tablespoon olive oil

1 garlic clove, minced

¼ teaspoon dried basil

¼ teaspoon dried oregano

1 (8-ounce) can tomato sauce

1 (17- to 18-ounce) tube cooked polenta

½ cup shredded mozzarella cheese

2 tablespoons freshly grated Parmesan cheese

In a skillet over medium-high heat, add the oil. Sauté the garlic, basil, and oregano for 30 to 60 seconds. Add the tomato sauce and bring to a boil. Reduce the heat and simmer for 10 to 15 minutes, or until thickened, stirring occasionally.

Meanwhile, set an oven rack in the second-closest setting to the broiler and preheat the broiler. Lightly coat a rimmed baking sheet with nonstick cooking spray.

Slice the polenta roll in half horizontally, and then cut each half lengthways into four "planks" (trim the rounded bit on the outside pieces so they can lie flat on the baking sheet). Place the polenta pieces on the baking sheet and broil for 4 to 5 minutes, or until the tops

begin to bubble and turn golden brown, checking every couple of minutes. Flip and broil for 3 to 5 minutes, or until golden brown and crispy on the edges.

Remove from the oven and top each plank with 1 tablespoon of tomato sauce, 1 tablespoon mozzarella cheese, and sprinkle with Parmesan. Broil for 1 to 2 minutes, or until the cheese has melted.

PER SERVING	
Calories	160
Fat	7 g
Saturated fat	2.5 g
Cholesterol	10 mg
Sodium	630 mg
Carbohydrate	20 g
Dietary fiber	4 g
Sugars	3 g
Protein	6 g
Calcium	150 mg
Potassium	230 mg

Peanut Noodles

These peanut noodles get an Asian spin from flavorful soy sauce, sesame oil, and fresh ginger. If you prefer a hotter, spicier dish, add a drop or two of chili oil or a pinch of red pepper flakes.

4 SERVINGS

4 ounces linguine, spaghetti, or soba noodles

¼ cup creamy peanut butter

2 tablespoons reduced-sodium soy sauce or tamari

2 tablespoons Asian sesame oil

1 tablespoon red wine vinegar or rice wine vinegar

1 tablespoon chopped fresh ginger

1 garlic clove, chopped

1 teaspoon honey, optional

Prepare the pasta according to package directions. After draining, rinse with cold water.

Meanwhile, in a blender, combine the peanut butter, soy sauce, sesame oil, vinegar, ginger, garlic, and honey, if desired, and blend until smooth.

In a bowl, combine the sauce and drained pasta and stir gently to incorporate. If the sauce is too thick, dilute with hot water, 1 tablespoon at a time.

PER SERVING

Calories	280
Fat	16 g
Saturated fat	2.5 g
Cholesterol	0 mg
Sodium	290 mg
Carbohydrate	26 g
Dietary fiber	2 g
Sugars	3 g
Protein	8 g
Calcium	20 mg
Potassium	150 mg

 TIP For added flavor and texture, top with chopped peanuts or julienned snow peas, bell peppers, or cucumber.

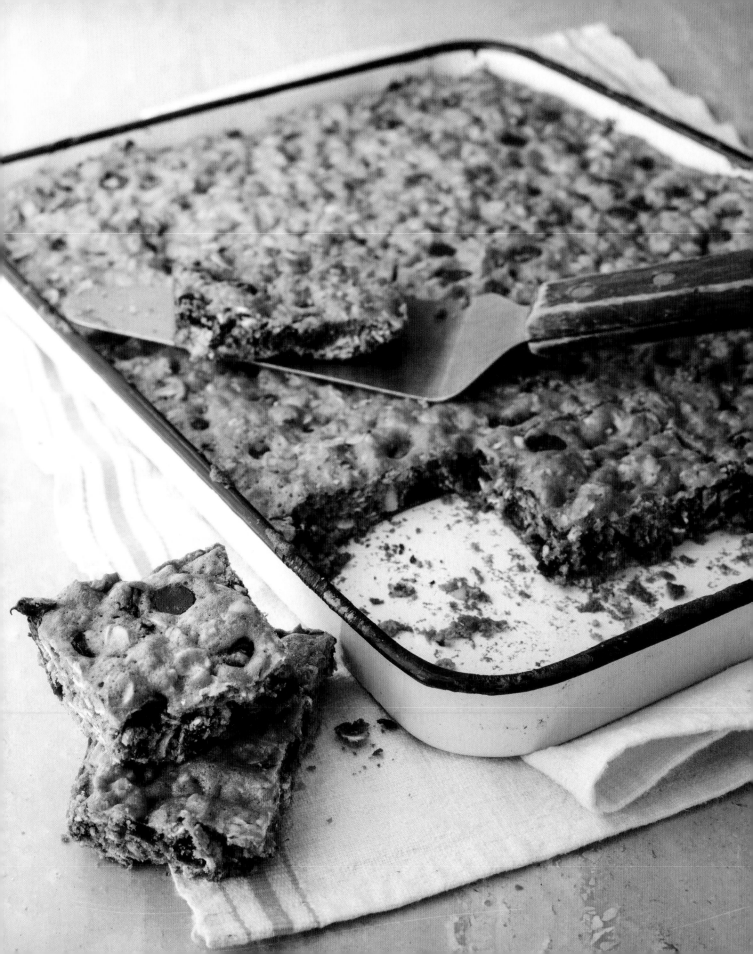

Chocolate Chip–Raisin Granola Bars

Although store-bought granola bars are marketed as "healthy," most commercial bars are so loaded with sugar and fat, it's hard to tell the difference between them and cookies. It's so much better for you to make your own with natural and healthful ingredients. You can even freeze the extras to have on hand when you want something a little sweet.

Don't despair that these bars will taste "too healthy." They still have your favorite ingredients: chocolate chips, raisins, and peanut butter, in addition to rolled oats, whole wheat flour, and very little oil.

Feel free to customize them by swapping your favorite dried fruit for the raisins and chopped nuts for the chips. The range of baking time allows you to bake to your preference: remove them from the oven earlier for a softer bar, or go a couple of minutes longer for crispier ones.

24 SERVINGS

1½ cups old-fashioned rolled oats

½ cup whole wheat flour

½ teaspoon baking soda

¼ teaspoon salt

2 tablespoons ground flaxseeds, optional

¾ cup raisins

¾ cup semisweet chocolate chips, preferably mini chips

2 eggs

¾ cup packed light brown sugar

½ cup chunky peanut butter

2 tablespoons canola oil

Preheat the oven to 350 degrees.

Line a 9-by-13-inch baking pan with aluminum foil and coat with nonstick cooking spray.

In a bowl, combine the oats, flour, baking soda, salt, and flaxseeds, if desired. Add the raisins and chocolate chips and stir to combine.

In a bowl, using an electric mixer, beat the eggs. Add the brown sugar and beat until smooth. Add the peanut butter and oil and beat until combined. On low speed, gradually add the dry ingredients until just combined, scraping down the beater(s) and sides to blend.

Spread the batter in the prepared pan; it will not be very thick. Using wet fingertips, evenly distribute the mixture.

Bake for 18 to 25 minutes, or until firm to the touch. Set the pan on a cooling rack to cool completely before cutting into squares.

PER SERVING

Calories	140
Fat	6 g
Saturated fat	2 g
Cholesterol	15 mg
Sodium	85 mg
Carbohydrate	20 g
Dietary fiber	2 g
Sugars	13 g
Protein	3 g
Calcium	20 mg
Potassium	130 mg

Cheesy French Toast

When you think of French toast, a sweet breakfast treat covered in syrup comes to mind. But in this savory version, the egg-soaked bread is coated with grated cheese, for a soft and satisfying small meal that's flavorful and rich without being overwhelming. You can use Cheddar or another distinctive cheese, such as Gruyère, or a combination of the two.

Another plus, this is a great way to use up leftover, stale bread. The drier the bread, the more liquid it will absorb, adding to its creamy, luscious texture.

Eat as is or top with scrambled eggs and arugula for a more substantial meal.

2 SERVINGS

1 egg

⅓ cup whole milk

Pinch or 2 dry mustard

2 (1-inch) slices hearty white or sourdough bread

½ teaspoon butter

½ cup (packed) grated Cheddar cheese

In a shallow bowl, beat the egg. Add the milk and mustard and whisk to combine.

Place the bread in the egg mixture and turn several times to coat (you may need to do each piece of bread separately).

In a skillet or griddle over medium heat, melt the butter. Top each slice of bread with 2 tablespoons of grated cheese, pressing it to adhere to the egg mixture. Carefully place the bread, cheese side down, in the skillet and cook until the bottoms are golden brown. Cover the tops with the remaining cheese, pressing to adhere, and carefully flip the bread.

Cook until the bottom is golden brown and the bread is heated through.

PER SERVING	
Calories	240
Fat	15 g
Saturated fat	8 g
Cholesterol	130 mg
Sodium	350 mg
Carbohydrate	13 g
Dietary fiber	0.5 g
Sugars	3 g
Protein	13 g
Calcium	280 mg
Potassium	140 mg

Peanut Butter–Banana–Chocolate Panini

Elvis should be smiling down on this sandwich, which blends sweet and savory while providing calories and nutrients. If you'd rather, Nutella (a creamy chocolate and hazelnut spread) is a perfect replacement for the chocolate chips in this sandwich. Just spread the peanut butter on one piece of bread, Nutella on the other, and sandwich the banana slices between them before grilling.

If you have a panini press, use it for making this sandwich. If not, just press the sandwich down with a spatula. If possible, cut one-inch slices from a hearty loaf of bakery-style white bread—the thicker bread will hold up better during cooking.

1 SERVING

2 tablespoons creamy peanut butter

2 tablespoons mini chocolate chips, 2 ounces finely chopped chocolate, or 2 tablespoons Nutella or other chocolate spread

2 (1-inch thick) slices sturdy white bread, egg bread, or other sliced bread

½ small ripe banana, thinly sliced

1 teaspoon butter, softened

In a bowl, combine the peanut butter and mini chocolate chips. Spread on one side of each piece of bread. Place banana on top of one slice of bread and top with the other slice, peanut butter side down. Spread the butter on the other sides of the bread. Place in a panini press or skillet over medium heat.

Cook until both sides are golden and the chocolate has melted, turning carefully and pressing the top of the sandwich firmly with a spatula if you are using a skillet.

PER SERVING	
Calories	850
Fat	37 g
Saturated fat	12 g
Cholesterol	90 mg
Sodium	820 mg
Carbohydrate	109 g
Dietary fiber	8 g
Sugars	23 g
Protein	24 g
Calcium	170 mg
Potassium	650 mg

TIP If bananas are unappealing, swirl raspberry jam or your favorite fruit spread into the peanut butter.

Grain Bowl with Spinach, Pickled Carrots, and Fried Egg

The dilemma: Is this dish "dinner for breakfast" or "breakfast for dinner"? Who cares? It's so good you'll crave it any time of the day.

The sky's the limit with this recipe: use whatever grain and leftover veggies you have on hand. If fried eggs aren't your thing, substitute a hard-boiled egg, sautéed tofu, chicken, or fish.

The miso-based dressing can easily be increased for larger groups or future meals. If you don't have miso, or if you are experiencing neutropenia and are advised not to consume miso paste, add a few shakes of soy sauce or salt to taste after combining the other ingredients.

1 SERVING

1 small carrot

2 tablespoons unseasoned rice wine vinegar, divided use

1 teaspoon granulated sugar

Salt

1 teaspoon white miso paste

1/2 teaspoon finely grated ginger

1/2 teaspoon honey

1/2 teaspoon toasted sesame oil

1 tablespoon canola oil

1 cup cooked quinoa, heated

1/4 avocado, thinly sliced

2 cups fresh baby spinach

1 egg

1/2 teaspoon sesame seeds, optional

Using a vegetable peeler, shave the carrot into very thin strips and place in a bowl. Add 1 tablespoon of the rice wine vinegar, sugar, and a pinch of salt and stir to combine. Set aside.

In a bowl, combine the remaining 1 tablespoon of rice wine vinegar, miso paste, ginger, honey, and sesame oil. Slowly add the canola oil, whisking to emulsify it. Set aside.

Place the quinoa in a bowl. Toss with half of the miso mixture. Place the avocado on top of the quinoa, covering one-quarter of the bowl. Set aside.

Lightly coat a nonstick skillet with nonstick cooking spray. Add the spinach and sauté until wilted. Place the spinach on top of the quinoa, covering one-quarter of the bowl. In the same skillet, cook the egg until it is set and not runny. Place the egg on top of the quinoa, covering one-quarter of the bowl. Cover the remaining quarter of the bowl with the pickled carrots, including the liquid. Drizzle the vegetables with the remaining dressing. Sprinkle with sesame seeds, if desired.

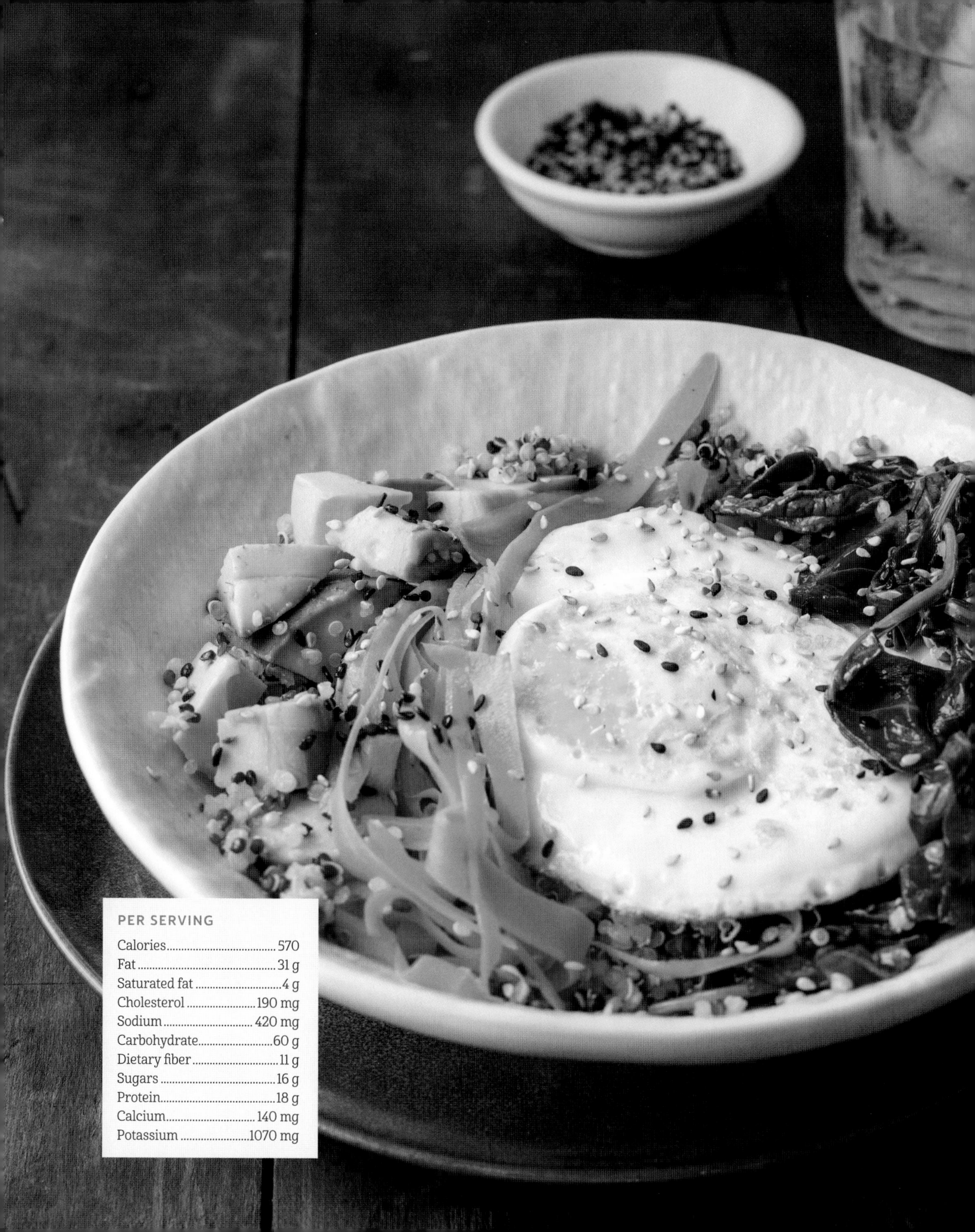

PER SERVING

Calories	570
Fat	31 g
Saturated fat	4 g
Cholesterol	190 mg
Sodium	420 mg
Carbohydrate	60 g
Dietary fiber	11 g
Sugars	16 g
Protein	18 g
Calcium	140 mg
Potassium	1070 mg

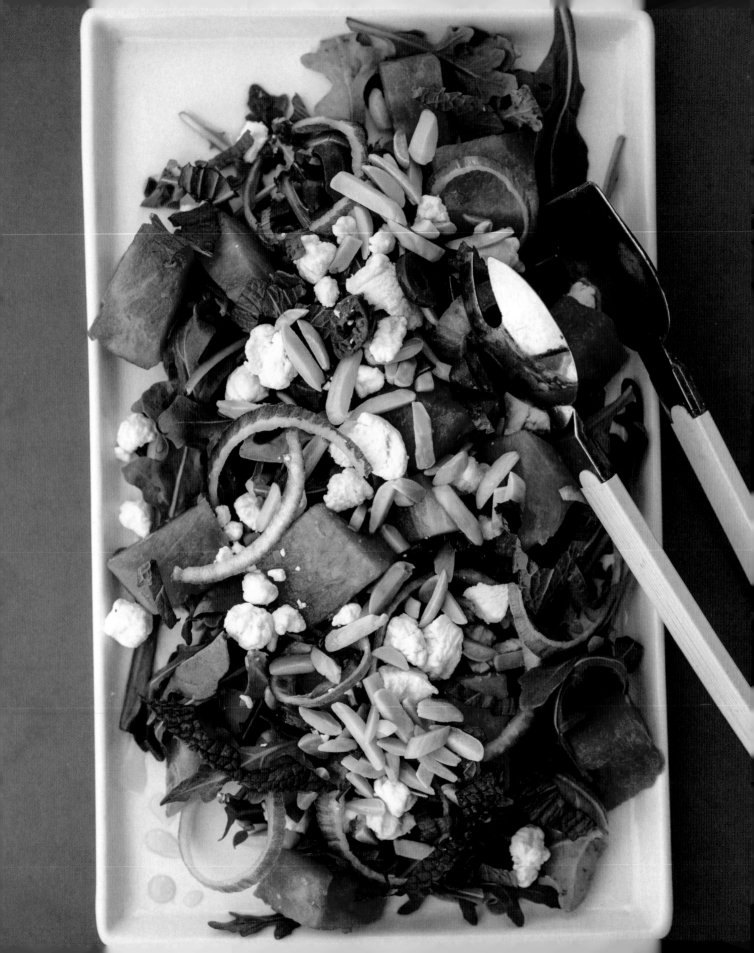

TC TASTE CHANGES

Rosemary Sweet and Spicy Nuts

Samosa Quesadillas

Gazpacho

Shrimp Puttanesca

Strawberry-Blueberry "Mocktail"

Tofu and Vegetable Red Curry

Lemon Chicken Sheet Pan Dinner

Southwest Bean Dip

Mulligatawny Soup

Beet-Horseradish Hummus

Mediterranean Egg and Tuna Pitas

Curried Chicken and Rice

Fusilli with Chicken, Leek, and Lemon

Tuna-Noodle Casserole with Lemon and Dill

Grilled Cheese and Cranberry Sandwich

Chickpea–Sweet Potato Curry

Vegetarian Roll-Up

Chai Latte

Arugula and Watermelon Salad

SOME TYPES OF TREATMENT MAY AFFECT YOUR SENSE OF TASTE. Chemotherapy, radiation therapy to the head and neck area, and certain medications may cause changes in the way you taste (and smell) food. When things don't taste or smell right or even have no taste or aroma at all, it can be difficult to get the calories and nutrition you need. You may find that food has a metallic, bitter, or even sour taste. Food may also taste too salty or sweet. Your old favorites may not be appealing or you may, surprisingly, develop a taste for something you did not like prior to treatment. Fortunately, changes in taste and smell usually resolve in a few months after treatment ends.

These tips can help manage changes in taste:

- If meat does not taste good, try eating other protein-rich foods such as eggs, dairy foods, or meatless options like beans or peas, tofu, seeds and nuts, and nut butters.

- Try marinating and cooking meat, poultry, or fish in naturally sweet juices; salad dressings; or barbecue, soy, or teriyaki sauce.

- To decrease metallic or bitter tastes, try adding a squeeze of lemon or lime juice or a splash of vinegar to vegetables or soups.

- Tart or sour foods like cranberries and pickled vegetables may offer more flavor.

- Foods with strong flavors, such as onion, garlic, and Parmesan cheese may cut through "blah" tastes.

- Fresh vegetables may be more appealing than canned or frozen ones.

- Fruit smoothies and frozen desserts such as sorbet or sherbet may be appealing.

- Try increasing the amounts of spice, herbs, or seasonings in recipes if it suits your tastes.

- Experiment with new foods or cuisines.

- Use plastic utensils instead of stainless flatware.

To keep your mouth clean, healthy, and tasting better, follow these daily mouth care suggestions:

- Be sure to brush your teeth and rinse your mouth after meals and snacks and before bed.

- Consider rinsing your mouth throughout the day with an easy-to-make homemade mouth rinse. Mix together four cups of water, one teaspoon of salt, and one teaspoon of baking soda. Swish the mixture in your mouth and then spit out.

CONTACT YOUR DOCTOR IN THESE SITUATIONS:

- Your mouth is sore or inflamed.

- You have open sores in your mouth.

- There are white patches on your tongue or on the inside of your mouth.

For more information about managing changes in taste or smell, visit the American Cancer Society website at cancer.org or call 800-227-2345.

Rosemary Sweet and Spicy Nuts

Nuts are a good protein source and handy on-the-go snack. While they are great eaten plain, coating them with a mixture of spices and aromatic chopped fresh rosemary leaves makes them even more enjoyable.

Suit your own flavor cravings by being a little generous with your seasonings. If you want more heat, up the cayenne or add a pinch or two of black pepper. Add a bit more brown sugar for something sweeter. If you want milder flavors, take it down a notch and use less.

The nuts may seem slightly soft after cooking, but they will continue to crisp up as they cool. Store extras in a zip-top bag or airtight container. They can also be frozen and taken out as needed. Defrost completely before eating.

12 SERVINGS

2 tablespoons chopped fresh rosemary leaves

2 tablespoons packed light brown sugar

1 teaspoon salt

1/4 teaspoon cayenne pepper

1 egg white

3 cups assorted unsalted nuts, such as cashews, almonds, walnuts, and/or pecans

Preheat the oven to 300 degrees. Line a rimmed baking sheet with parchment paper.

In a bowl, combine the rosemary, brown sugar, salt, and cayenne pepper.

In a medium bowl, beat the egg white until frothy. Add the nuts and stir well to coat. Add the spice mixture and stir well to coat.

Spread the nuts in a single layer on the parchment. Bake for 18 to 22 minutes, stirring once, or until golden brown and fragrant. Cool on the baking sheet.

PER SERVING (ABOUT 1/4 CUP)	
Calories	210
Fat	18 g
Saturated fat	2 g
Cholesterol	0 mg
Sodium	170 mg
Carbohydrate	9 g
Dietary fiber	2 g
Sugars	4 g
Protein	5 g
Calcium	40 mg
Potassium	180 mg

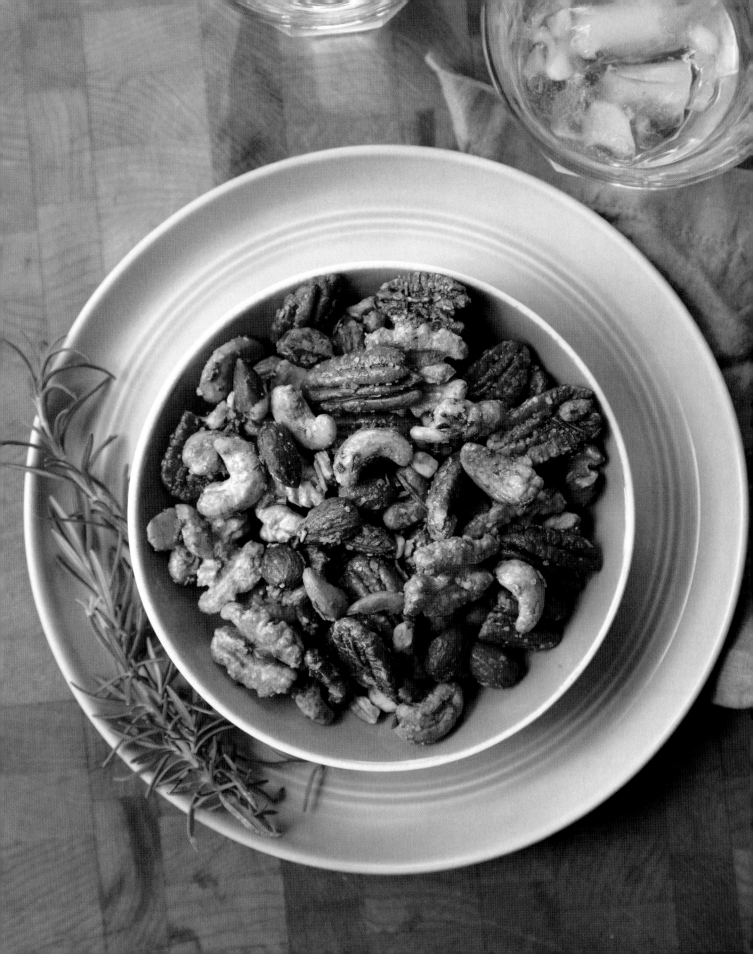

Samosa Quesadillas

An Indian cuisine-inspired vegetable and spice mixture provides warming notes to this untraditional quesadilla. Normally samosas are fried in a pastry crust; using tortillas makes preparation so much easier.

It you have a sore mouth, lessen or omit the spices from the filling and serve it "unstuffed" as a soft entrée. If you want more zest, double the garam masala and coriander.

4 SERVINGS

8 ounces Yukon Gold or other white potatoes, peeled and quartered

8 ounces sweet potatoes, peeled and cut into 1-inch pieces

1 tablespoon canola oil

1 small onion, finely chopped

2 garlic cloves, minced

1/4 teaspoon garam masala

1/4 teaspoon ground coriander

1/2 cup frozen peas

1/4 cup finely chopped fresh cilantro

Salt

4 ounces goat cheese, crumbled

8 (8-inch) whole wheat tortillas

1 cup (4 ounces) shredded Cheddar cheese

Preheat the oven to 300 degrees.

In a saucepan, combine the white and sweet potatoes and cover with water. Bring to a boil, reduce the heat, partially cover, and simmer for 15 minutes, or until the potatoes are very tender. Drain the potatoes and set aside

Meanwhile, in a skillet over medium heat, add the oil. Sauté the onion for 5 minutes, or until softened. Add the garlic, garam masala, and coriander to the skillet and sauté for 1 minute, or until fragrant. Add the peas, reserved potatoes, and cilantro and stir to combine, mashing the potatoes to incorporate them. Season with salt.

Divide the goat cheese on four tortillas, top with the vegetable mixture, and sprinkle with

Cheddar cheese. Top with remaining tortillas.

Lightly coat a nonstick skillet with nonstick cooking spray and place over medium heat. Add the quesadillas one at a time and cook for 1 to 2 minutes per side, or until crisp on the outside and warm throughout. Transfer to a baking sheet to keep warm in the oven while cooking the remaining quesadillas.

PER SERVING	
Calories	650
Fat	30 g
Saturated fat	16 g
Cholesterol	60 mg
Sodium	840 mg
Carbohydrate	73 g
Dietary fiber	14 g
Sugars	8 g
Protein	25 g
Calcium	530 mg
Potassium	650 mg

TIP If you are experiencing neutropenia, substitute mild Cheddar or Monterey Jack for the goat cheese.

Gazpacho

This chilled soup is filled with healthy vegetables and provides nutrients and bright flavor in a bowl. To speed prep time, use a food processor for chopping your vegetables and mixing. You may need to do this step in two or more batches, depending on the size of your food processor. To chop the vegetables (without pulverizing them), use the pulse button. The vegetables can also be chopped by hand.

This recipe may not be appropriate for those who are experiencing gas.

10 SERVINGS

1 large garlic clove

1 small (or 1/2 large) red onion, cut into 1- to 2-inch pieces

1 green bell pepper, seeded and cut into 1- to 2-inch pieces

1 red bell pepper, seeded and cut into 1- to 2-inch pieces

1 cucumber, peeled, seeded, and cut into 1- to 2-inch pieces

1 (28-ounce) can Italian plum tomatoes

2 tablespoons olive oil

2 tablespoons red wine vinegar

2 teaspoons salt

1 teaspoon granulated sugar

1/2 teaspoon ground black pepper

Tabasco or other hot red pepper sauce

2 cups tomato juice or tomato-vegetable juice

In a food processor, with the motor running, drop in the garlic and purée. Stop the machine, add the onion, and pulse until coarsely chopped. Add both bell peppers and cucumber and pulse until coarsely chopped. Add the tomatoes, oil, vinegar, salt, sugar, black pepper, and a few shakes of Tabasco and pulse until all of the vegetables are chopped but still chunky, about 30 seconds. Do not overprocess.

Transfer to a large bowl. Add the tomato juice and stir to combine. Cover and refrigerate for at least 2 hours before serving.

PER SERVING	
Calories	60
Fat	3 g
Saturated fat	0 g
Cholesterol	0 mg
Sodium	870 mg
Carbohydrate	10 g
Dietary fiber	2 g
Sugars	6 g
Protein	2 g
Calcium	40 mg
Potassium	350 mg

TIP Canned tomatoes are better than fresh tomatoes as a source of the antioxidant lycopene.

Shrimp Puttanesca

When your taste buds need a little resuscitation, try this salty, spicy shrimp dish. Olives, capers, and anchovies add brininess, and garlic and red pepper flakes provide intensity. Start with these amounts and adjust ingredients to taste if you are craving salt or want more heat. Enjoy on its own or serve with a grain or pasta of your choice.

4 SERVINGS

2 tablespoons olive oil

3 garlic cloves, thinly sliced

1/4 teaspoon red pepper flakes

1 pound shrimp, shelled and deveined and patted dry

1 (14.5-ounce) can diced tomatoes

1 teaspoon anchovy paste or 1 anchovy fillet, drained and chopped

1/2 teaspoon dried oregano

1/2 teaspoon dried basil

2 tablespoons capers

1/4 cup chopped Kalamata olives

Salt and freshly ground black pepper

In a large skillet over medium-high heat, add the oil. Sauté the garlic and red pepper flakes for 1 minute. Add the shrimp and cook for 1 minute per side without stirring. Remove the shrimp and set aside.

In the same skillet, add the tomatoes and their juice, anchovy paste, oregano, and basil and bring to a boil. Reduce the heat and simmer for 10 minutes, or until thickened, stirring occasionally. Add the capers and olives and simmer for 1 minute. Return the shrimp to the skillet and sauté for 1 minute, or until the shrimp is heated through. Season with salt and pepper.

PER SERVING

Calories	170
Fat	10 g
Saturated fat	1 g
Cholesterol	120 mg
Sodium	580 mg
Carbohydrate	6 g
Dietary fiber	1 g
Sugars	3 g
Protein	17 g
Calcium	100 mg
Potassium	380 mg

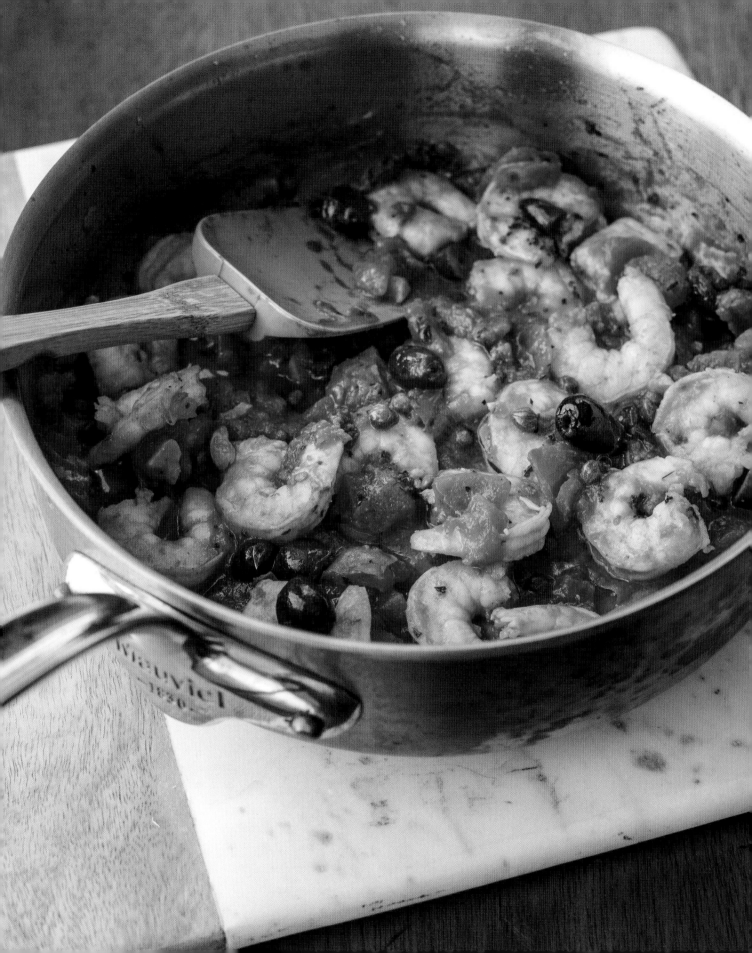

Strawberry-Blueberry "Mocktail"

When you feel like a little pick-me-up, try this effervescent fruity concoction. Sparkling apple cider feels special and festive but is appropriate to sip on throughout the day, unlike some other bubbly beverages. Instead of adding seltzer for fizz, try sparkling apple cider, which boosts other flavors instead of diluting them. If you feel like a less intense drink, then by all means use carbonated water.

Choose any berry or combination or use defrosted frozen mixed berries for a medley of flavors.

2 SERVINGS

½ cup fresh or frozen
   strawberries, defrosted

½ cup fresh or frozen
   blueberries, defrosted

1 cup sparkling apple cider

Ice, optional

In a blender, combine the strawberries and blueberries and blend until smooth. Strain the mixture into a container or bowl, pushing down with a spoon to extract all the liquid. Divide the purée between two glasses and fill with sparkling cider. Add ice, if desired.

PER SERVING	
Calories	90
Fat	0 g
Saturated fat	0 g
Cholesterol	0 mg
Sodium	0 mg
Carbohydrate	22 g
Dietary fiber	0.5 g
Sugars	20 g
Protein	0 g
Calcium	10 mg
Potassium	100 mg

 TIP Sparkling apple cider comes in a champagne-like bottle. Once opened, keep it well sealed to maintain the carbonation.

Tofu and Vegetable Red Curry

This Thai classic is easy to prepare at home using premade curry paste and canned coconut milk. If you don't care for tofu, you can substitute chicken, shrimp, salmon, or a lean cut of beef.

If your taste buds are a little flat, try a squeeze of lime at the end of cooking. If you crave salt, add another teaspoon of fish sauce; more sweetness, a bit more brown sugar. For added calories, use full-fat coconut milk and stir a couple of tablespoons of peanut butter into the sauce. If weight gain is an issue, choose light coconut milk.

4 SERVINGS

1 (16-ounce) block extra firm tofu

1 tablespoon canola oil

1 red bell pepper, seeded and thinly sliced

2 cups (5 to 7 ounces) sliced white mushrooms

2 cups (5 to 7 ounces) snap or snow peas

3 tablespoons red curry paste

1 (13.5-ounce) can coconut milk, well shaken

1 to 2 tablespoons light or dark brown sugar

1 to 2 tablespoons fish sauce

1 cinnamon stick

1/2 cup frozen peas

2 tablespoons sliced fresh basil leaves

1 lime, cut into four wedges, optional

Line a plate with paper towels and place the tofu on top. Cover with paper towels and top with another plate weighed down with cans or a heavy pot for 30 minutes to release excess water. Pat dry and cut into 1/2-inch cubes.

In a large, preferably nonstick, skillet over medium-high heat, add the oil. Cook the tofu for 1 to 2 minutes per side, or until golden. Remove the tofu and set aside.

In the same skillet, sauté the bell pepper, mushrooms, and snap peas for 3 to 5 minutes, or until just softened. Remove and add to the tofu.

In the same skillet, add the curry paste and stir for a few seconds, or until fragrant. Add

the coconut milk, 1 tablespoon of the brown sugar, 1 tablespoon of the fish sauce, and the cinnamon stick and stir to combine. Bring to a boil, reduce the heat, and simmer for 15 minutes, or until reduced by about half. Add the reserved tofu mixture and the peas and sauté for 3 to 5 minutes, or until heated through. Taste and add brown sugar and/or fish sauce, if desired. Garnish with basil. Serve with a wedge of lime to squeeze on the dish, if desired.

PER SERVING	
Calories	270
Fat	16 g
Saturated fat	6 g
Cholesterol	0 mg
Sodium	810 mg
Carbohydrate	18 g
Dietary fiber	4 g
Sugars	9 g
Protein	18 g
Calcium	260 mg
Potassium	700 mg

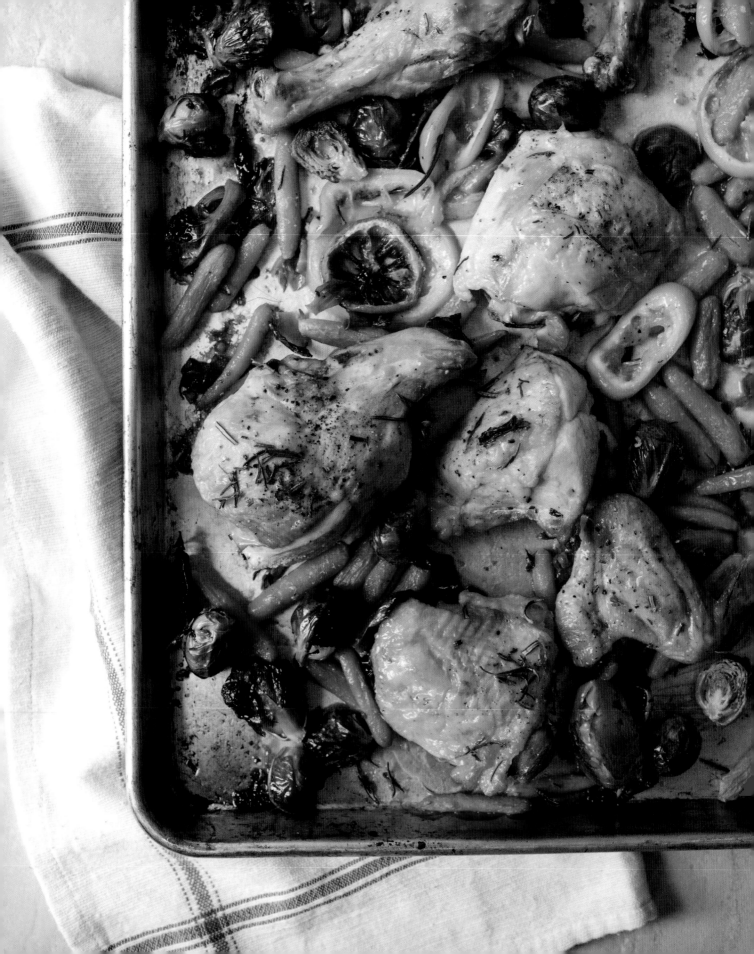

Lemon Chicken Sheet Pan Dinner

Sheet pan dinners make mealtime easier; the protein and vegetables cook together, making cleanup a breeze. (Make it even quicker by lining the baking sheets with foil or parchment.) The roasted lemon slices provide acidity for those craving sharper flavors.

Add a side of brown rice, quinoa, or farro and you're all set.

8 SERVINGS

1 pound baby carrots

1 pound Brussels sprouts, trimmed

2 lemons, cut into thin slices

2 tablespoons olive oil, divided use

Salt and freshly ground black pepper

1 whole (3½- to 4-pound) chicken, cut into 10 pieces (breasts double cut)

2 teaspoons chopped fresh rosemary leaves or 1 teaspoon dried rosemary

Preheat the oven to 425 degrees. Lightly coat two rimmed baking sheets with nonstick cooking spray. Top with the carrots, Brussels sprouts, and lemon slices, dividing the vegetables evenly between the baking sheets. Drizzle with 1 tablespoon of the oil, sprinkle with salt and pepper, and stir to combine. Place the chicken on top, dividing it evenly between the baking sheets. Drizzle with the remaining 1 tablespoon of oil and sprinkle the chicken and vegetables with the rosemary, salt, and pepper.

Bake for 20 minutes, stir the vegetables, and bake for 25 minutes, or until the chicken is cooked through and the vegetables are tender.

PER SERVING

Calories	260
Fat	14 g
Saturated fat	3.5 g
Cholesterol	70 mg
Sodium	120 mg
Carbohydrate	10 g
Dietary fiber	3 g
Sugars	4 g
Protein	23 g
Calcium	50 mg
Potassium	550 mg

Southwest Bean Dip

This dip satisfies a craving for southwestern flavor but is still fine for a sensitive mouth. It has just enough chili powder to add spice without being too strong. Serve with soft tortillas or pita if your mouth is sensitive or carrot sticks and bell pepper strips for added fiber. Garnish with fresh cilantro if you have some on hand.

Refrigerate for thirty minutes before serving to allow flavors to meld.

6 SERVINGS

1 garlic clove

1 (15-ounce) can cannellini beans, rinsed and drained

Juice of 1 lime

2 tablespoons olive oil

1½ teaspoons chili powder

½ teaspoon ground cumin

¼ teaspoon salt

In a food processor, with the motor running, drop in the garlic and purée. Stop the machine, add the beans, half of the lime juice, the oil, chili powder, cumin, and salt, and process until smooth. Taste and add more lime juice, seasonings, or salt, if needed.

PER SERVING

Calories	90
Fat	5 g
Saturated fat	0.5 g
Cholesterol	0 mg
Sodium	140 mg
Carbohydrate	10 g
Dietary fiber	3 g
Sugars	0 g
Protein	4 g
Calcium	20 mg
Potassium	180 mg

 TIP Cannellini beans are also known as white kidney beans.

Mulligatawny Soup

This curried chicken soup, richly flavored with apples, lemon, and cloves, was originally prepared by Indian cooks for British colonialists. They took the recipe back to England and then later introduced it in the United States. Its interplay of flavors will have your tongue singing.

10 SERVINGS

2 tablespoons canola oil

1 carrot, chopped

1 onion, chopped

1 celery stalk, chopped

1 Granny Smith apple, peeled, cored, and chopped

2 tablespoons all-purpose flour

1 tablespoon curry powder

1/8 teaspoon ground cloves

6 cups homemade chicken broth (page 40) or store-bought reduced-sodium broth

1 (14.5-ounce) can diced tomatoes, drained, or 1 ripe tomato, chopped

1 tablespoon fresh lemon juice

1/2 cup white rice

1 pound boneless chicken breasts, cut into 1/2-inch pieces

Salt and freshly ground black pepper

In a stockpot over medium-high heat, add the oil. Sauté the carrot, onion, celery, and apple for 8 to 10 minutes, or until softened. Add the flour, curry, and cloves and cook for 1 to 2 minutes, stirring constantly. Add the broth, tomatoes, and lemon juice and stir to combine. Bring to a boil. Add the rice and stir to combine. Reduce the heat, partially cover, and simmer for 10 minutes, stirring occasionally.

Add the chicken and cook for 5 to 10 minutes, or until the chicken and rice are cooked through. Season with salt and pepper.

PER SERVING

Calories	150
Fat	4 g
Saturated fat	0.5 g
Cholesterol	25 mg
Sodium	380 mg
Carbohydrate	15 g
Dietary fiber	1 g
Sugars	4 g
Protein	12 g
Calcium	40 mg
Potassium	320 mg

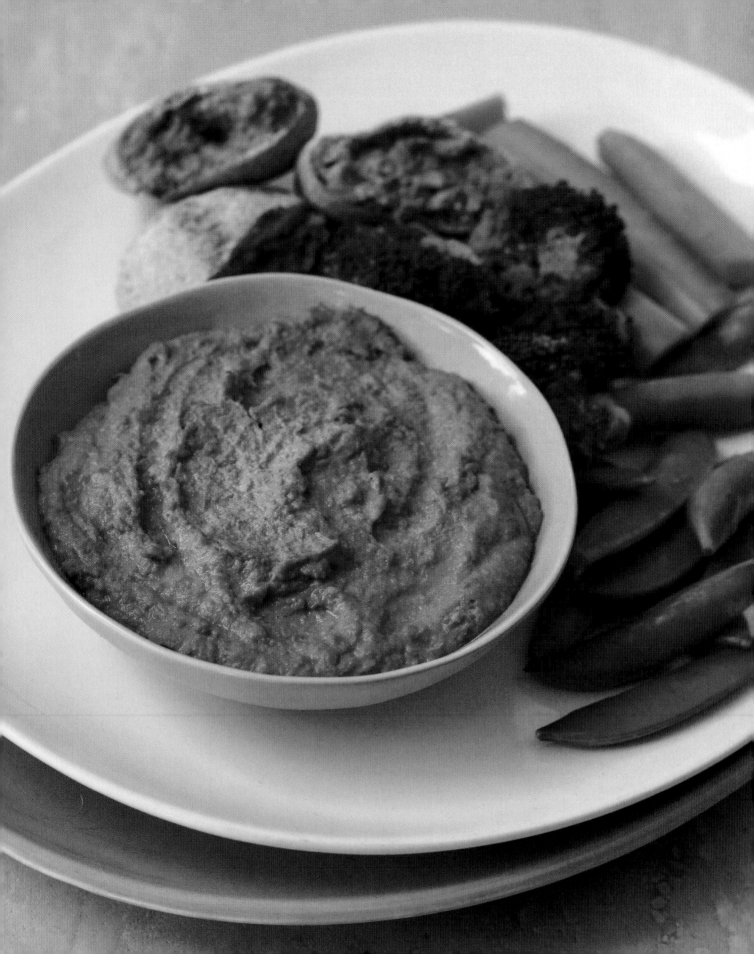

Beet-Horseradish Hummus

Hummus goes from dull to vibrant with the addition of a cooked beet. Not only do beets taste great and add a visual boost, they provide potassium, fiber, and vitamin C. If you need a bit more zing to activate your appetite, up the horseradish, salt, or lemon juice.

Tahini is a paste made from ground sesame seeds. Because the oil separates, make sure to stir it well before using. Look for it in the international food aisle of your supermarket.

This spread is also a good choice if you are having trouble swallowing. If you need to change the consistency, thin with water or lemon juice. If you are experiencing mouth sores, omit the citrus and horseradish.

You can buy packaged cooked beets in the produce section, use canned beets, or cook your own: simply wrap the beet in foil and bake for an hour at 400 degrees.

8 SERVINGS

2 garlic cloves

1 cooked beet, quartered

1 (15-ounce) can chickpeas, rinsed and drained

2 tablespoons tahini

3 to 5 tablespoons fresh lemon juice

2 tablespoons hot water

2 tablespoons olive oil

1 to 2 tablespoons prepared horseradish

1/2 to 1 teaspoon salt

In a food processor, pulse the garlic until finely chopped. Add the beet and process until smooth. Add the chickpeas, tahini, 3 tablespoons of the lemon juice, water, oil, 1 tablespoon of the horseradish, and 1/2 teaspoon of the salt. Process until smooth, scraping down the blade and sides to blend. Taste and add lemon juice, horseradish, or salt, if desired.

PER SERVING

Calories	110
Fat	6 g
Saturated fat	1 g
Cholesterol	0 mg
Sodium	220 mg
Carbohydrate	11 g
Dietary fiber	3 g
Sugars	2 g
Protein	4 g
Calcium	40 mg
Potassium	140 mg

Mediterranean Egg and Tuna Pitas

This sandwich combines the flavors of two French classic dishes, salade niçoise and pan-bagnat, which complement each other so well in this incarnation.

If you prefer stronger tuna flavor, choose chunk light instead of white. For even stronger Mediterranean flavor, add sliced black olives or olive spread.

To give the shallots time to soften and "pickle," let them sit for at least an hour.

2 SERVINGS

1/4 cup white wine vinegar

2 tablespoons granulated sugar

2 shallots or 1/2 red onion, very thinly sliced

3 tablespoons fresh lemon juice

2 tablespoons chopped fresh dill

1 tablespoon extra virgin olive oil

1/2 teaspoon Dijon mustard

1 (5-ounce) can solid white tuna, drained

1 tablespoon capers

5 grape tomatoes, chopped

Salt and freshly ground black pepper

1 whole wheat pita, cut in half

2 hard-boiled eggs, peeled and sliced

1/2 cup arugula

In a bowl, combine the vinegar and sugar. Add the shallots and stir to combine. Set aside for 1 hour or more, stirring occasionally, until the shallots are softened and have mellowed. Drain shallots from the liquid before using.

When shallots are ready, in a bowl, combine the lemon juice, dill, olive oil, and mustard. Add the tuna and stir to combine. Add the capers and tomatoes and gently stir to combine. Season with salt and pepper.

In each pita half, place slices of egg. Top with a layer of tuna, shallots, and arugula.

PER SERVING	
Calories	330
Fat	14 g
Saturated fat	3 g
Cholesterol	210 mg
Sodium	620 mg
Carbohydrate	28 g
Dietary fiber	4 g
Sugars	6 g
Protein	24 g
Calcium	70 mg
Potassium	440 mg

Curried Chicken and Rice

This fragrant curry dish provides a lot of flavor without being overpowering. If you're new to curry, use two tablespoons curry powder as indicated; if you want more intense flavor, three tablespoons will do it.

Because the rice and chicken cook together, simply add a green salad to round out the meal.

For easy cleanup, cook in a baking dish that can go from stovetop to oven to table.

8 SERVINGS

1 whole (3 ½- to 4-pound) chicken, cut into 10 pieces (breasts double cut)

Salt and freshly ground black pepper

3 tablespoons canola oil

1 onion, chopped

2 garlic cloves, finely chopped

1 ½ cups basmati rice

2 tablespoons curry powder

1 teaspoon ground cumin

½ teaspoon ground ginger or 1 teaspoon finely chopped fresh ginger

½ teaspoon red pepper flakes, optional

3 cups homemade chicken broth (page 40) or store-bought reduced-sodium broth

½ cup golden raisins or brown raisins

½ cup slivered almonds, toasted

Preheat the oven to 350 degrees.

Sprinkle the chicken with salt and pepper.

In a large ovenproof skillet over medium-high heat, add the oil. Brown the chicken for 3 to 5 minutes per side. Remove the chicken and set aside. (You may need to brown the chicken in two or more batches, depending on the size of your skillet.)

Reduce the heat to medium and add the onion to the skillet. Sauté for 3 to 5 minutes, or until softened. Add the garlic and sauté for 1 minute. Add the rice, curry powder, cumin, ginger, and red pepper flakes, if desired, and stir to combine. Add the broth and bring to a boil, scraping up any browned bits clinging to the pan. Return the chicken to the skillet and cover.

Bake for 30 to 40 minutes, or until the rice is tender, the broth has been absorbed, and the chicken is cooked through. Just before serving, add the raisins and almonds.

PER SERVING

Calories	450
Fat	21 g
Saturated fat	4 g
Cholesterol	71 mg
Sodium	250 mg
Carbohydrate	37 g
Dietary fiber	2 g
Sugars	7 g
Protein	27 g
Calcium	60 mg
Potassium	360 mg

TIP Most supermarkets sell chicken cut into eight pieces. Cut the breasts in half for ten total pieces.

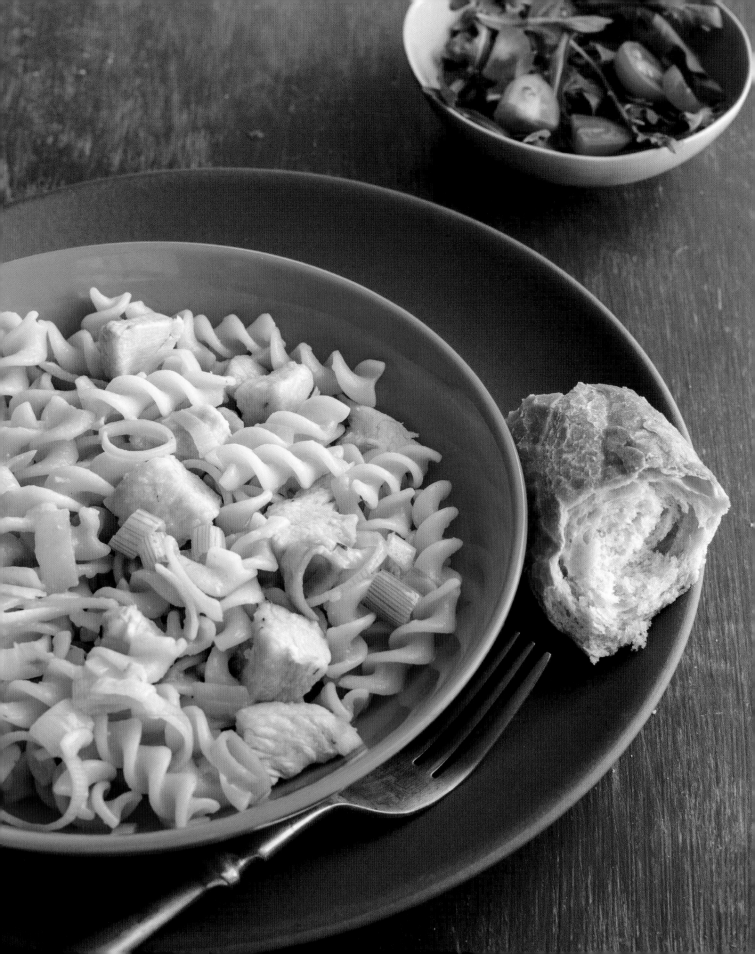

Fusilli with Chicken, Leek, and Lemon

Acidity brightens a dish, making it more appealing if your taste buds are having trouble finding something to tempt them. This chicken and pasta combo in a light lemon sauce benefits from a generous amount of citrus.

When making a pan sauce such as this one, don't use a nonstick pan or worry about ingredients sticking to the pan a bit during cooking (although you don't want them to burn). The flour and bits of vegetables that adhere to the pan are incorporated into the sauce to thicken it and add flavor. The corkscrew shape of the pasta helps hold the sauce.

Season with added salt or lemon juice to taste during the final moments.

4 SERVINGS

8 ounces fusilli or other shaped pasta

1/4 cup flour

1 teaspoon dried oregano

Salt and freshly ground black pepper

1 pound boneless, skinless chicken breasts, cut into 3/4-inch pieces

1 to 2 tablespoons olive oil

1 leek, white and light green parts only, thickly sliced

2 garlic cloves, minced

1 cup homemade chicken broth (page 40) or store-bought reduced-sodium broth

1 lemon, zested and juiced

Prepare the pasta according to the package directions for al dente (just firm). Drain and set aside.

Meanwhile, in a bowl, combine the flour and oregano and sprinkle with salt and pepper. Add the chicken and turn to coat.

In a large skillet over medium heat, add 1 tablespoon of the oil. Sauté the leek for 5 minutes, or until softened. Add the garlic and sauté for 1 minute. Remove and set aside. Add the chicken and cook for 2 to 3 minutes per side, or until lightly golden brown and cooked through, adding the remaining 1 tablespoon of oil if necessary. Remove the chicken and add to the leek.

In the same skillet, add the broth and bring to a boil for 3 to 5 minutes, or until reduced by half, stirring frequently to dislodge any bits of food that might have stuck to the bottom of the skillet. Reduce the heat to medium-low, return the reserved chicken and leek, pasta, lemon zest, and lemon juice and sauté for 1 to 2 minutes, or until the chicken is heated through and coated with sauce. Season with salt and pepper.

PER SERVING

Calories	400
Fat	7 g
Saturated fat	1.5 g
Cholesterol	65 mg
Sodium	190 mg
Carbohydrate	50 g
Dietary fiber	3 g
Sugars	3 g
Protein	32 g
Calcium	50 mg
Potassium	390 mg

Tuna-Noodle Casserole with Lemon and Dill

This made-from-scratch version of the classic American dish gets vibrancy from fresh herbs and citrus. If you are craving protein, add another can of tuna. For more pronounced citrus flavor, grate extra lemon zest over the topping after cooking.

6 SERVINGS

6 ounces egg noodles

2 tablespoons canola oil, divided use

1 onion, finely chopped

1 stalk celery, finely chopped

8 ounces white mushrooms, sliced

2 garlic cloves, minced

¼ cup white wine, optional

3 tablespoons butter

3 tablespoons all-purpose flour

1 cup homemade chicken broth (page 40) or store-bought reduced-sodium broth

1 cup milk

1 (5-ounce) can solid white tuna, drained and flaked

1 cup frozen peas

¼ cup chopped fresh dill

Zest of 1 lemon

Salt and freshly ground pepper

1 ½ cups fresh bread crumbs or panko

1 packed cup grated Cheddar cheese

Preheat the oven to 375 degrees. Lightly coat an 8-by-8-inch (or other 1½-quart) baking pan with nonstick cooking spray.

Boil the noodles for 4 to 5 minutes, or until very al dente. Drain, rinse with cold water, drain again, and set aside.

In a large skillet over medium-high heat, add 1 tablespoon of the oil. Add the onion and celery and sauté for 5 to 8 minutes, or until softened. Add the mushrooms and garlic and sauté for 5 minutes, or until the mushrooms soften and release their liquid. Add the wine, if desired, and bring to a boil. Cook until it evaporates, stirring frequently. Remove from the heat and set aside.

Meanwhile, in a saucepan over medium-low heat, melt the butter. Add the flour and whisk constantly for 1 minute to incorporate. When the mixture turns golden, gradually add the broth and bring to a boil, whisking constantly. Add the milk and simmer for 2 to 3 minutes, or until thickened and smooth, whisking frequently. Add the tuna, peas, dill, vegetable mixture, lemon zest, and reserved pasta and stir to combine. Season with salt and pepper. Transfer to the baking pan.

In a bowl, combine the bread crumbs and cheese. Drizzle with the remaining 1 tablespoon of oil and stir to combine. Sprinkle the mixture over the casserole. Bake for 20 to 30 minutes, or until the topping is golden brown.

PER SERVING	
Calories	410
Fat	21 g
Saturated fat	10 g
Cholesterol	75 mg
Sodium	430 mg
Carbohydrate	38 g
Dietary fiber	3 g
Sugars	7 g
Protein	19 g
Calcium	230 mg
Potassium	420 mg

Grilled Cheese and Cranberry Sandwich

This combination of sweet and savory helps combat the metallic taste that can be a side effect of some treatments. Stonewall Kitchen, Sarabeth's, and Wild Thyme brands all make versions of cranberry relish or jam, or you can use the Cranberry-Pear Compote on page 142.

Using mayonnaise instead of butter when making grilled cheese has a couple of advantages: it is easy to spread and it has a higher smoke point than butter, making it less likely to burn before the cheese has fully melted.

1 SERVING

½ teaspoon mayonnaise

2 slices rye, whole wheat, or other hearty bread

2 tablespoons cranberry relish or jam

2 ounces sharp Cheddar cheese, thinly sliced or shredded

Spread the mayonnaise on one side of each piece of bread and place them on a plate, mayonnaise side down. Spread the upturned slices with the cranberry relish. Top one slice of the bread with the cheese. Top with the remaining slice of bread, cranberry relish side facing down.

In a skillet over medium heat, carefully place the sandwich. Cook until the bottom is golden brown and the cheese begins to melt, pressing down with a spatula to help the melted cheese adhere to the bread. Carefully turn the sandwich, and cook until the bottom is golden brown and the cheese has melted, pressing down with the spatula occasionally.

PER SERVING

Calories	440
Fat	23 g
Saturated fat	12 g
Cholesterol	55 mg
Sodium	780 mg
Carbohydrate	40 g
Dietary fiber	4 g
Sugars	9 g
Protein	20 g
Calcium	490 mg
Potassium	160 mg

 TIP If you are experiencing neutropenia, substitute mild Cheddar or Monterey Jack for the sharp Cheddar.

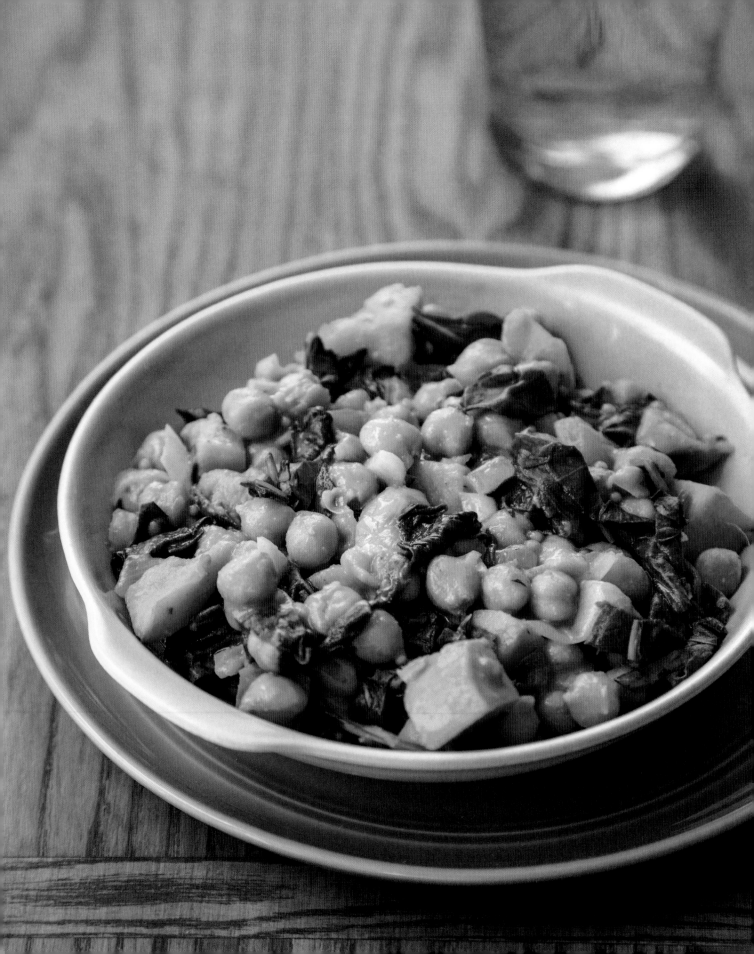

Chickpea–Sweet Potato Curry

This coconut-curry sauce isn't overpowering but provides distinctive flavor when you are experiencing taste changes.

For an even stronger flavor profile, feel free to substitute more assertive greens, such as thinly sliced kale, Swiss chard, or mustard greens for the spinach. Because heartier greens will take longer to cook, add them when you add the coconut milk.

Either full-fat or light coconut milk will work in this dish, so choose the option that's best for you. If you need to add calories, go for full-fat; if not, light will be equally delicious.

4 SERVINGS

1 tablespoon canola oil

1 onion, chopped

1 (8- to 10-ounce) sweet potato, peeled and cut into 1/2-inch pieces

2 garlic cloves, minced

1 tablespoon finely chopped fresh ginger

2 teaspoons curry powder

1 teaspoon mustard seeds

1 teaspoon ground coriander

1 1/2 cups unsweetened coconut milk, well shaken

1/2 cup water

1 (15-ounce) can chickpeas, rinsed and drained

1 (5- to 6-ounce) package fresh baby spinach

Salt and freshly ground black pepper

In a skillet over medium-high heat, add the oil. Sauté the onion and sweet potato for 3 to 5 minutes, or until the onion softens. Add the garlic and ginger and sauté for 1 minute. Add the curry powder, mustard seeds, and coriander and sauté for 30 seconds, or until fragrant. Add the coconut milk and water and bring to a boil, stirring to combine. Reduce the heat, cover, and simmer for 20 minutes, or until the sweet potato is tender. Add the chickpeas and stir to combine. Add the spinach a handful at a time, stirring until wilted. Season with salt and pepper.

PER SERVING	
Calories	270
Fat	11 g
Saturated fat	5 g
Cholesterol	0 mg
Sodium	170 mg
Carbohydrate	35 g
Dietary fiber	8 g
Sugars	9 g
Protein	10 g
Calcium	120 mg
Potassium	790 mg

Vegetarian Roll-Up

When you just want small bites, make a roll-up sandwich and slice off enough for a little meal when hunger strikes. This way, you'll always have something ready to eat when you feel like it. Cover leftovers with plastic wrap.

Adding an herbed or flavored cheese is a tasty way to add zing and calories. Choose any variety you like; Havarti with dill and Cheddar with horseradish are both good options. An herbed soft cheese spread, such as Boursin Garlic & Fine Herb, also can be used. For a blander taste, choose a plain cheese. If you're experiencing neutropenia, be sure to use a pasteurized cheese spread.

Sprinkle extra veggies, such as shredded carrots, for added fiber and nutrition.

1 SERVING

2 large slices (about 2 ounces) Havarti with dill or plain Havarti cheese

1 (8-inch) whole wheat or plain flour tortilla or flatbread such as lavash

10 to 15 fresh spinach or arugula leaves

⅓ ripe avocado, chopped

⅓ cup roasted red pepper, patted dry and chopped

Place the cheese over the tortilla to cover. Microwave for 45 to 60 seconds on high, or until cheese melts. Layer the spinach, avocado, and roasted red pepper on top of the tortilla. Roll up jellyroll style. Slice into 2-inch pieces.

PER SERVING

Calories	490
Fat	30 g
Saturated fat	14 g
Cholesterol	40 mg
Sodium	990 mg
Carbohydrate	37 g
Dietary fiber	7 g
Sugars	4 g
Protein	18 g
Calcium	480 mg
Potassium	580 mg

Chai Latte

This milky tea drink is flavored with aromatic spices that are calming to the stomach. It's a coffeehouse favorite that is easy to prepare at home.

A small seedpod, cardamom is a spice that is often used in baking and in Indian cuisine. It is available in spice markets, specialty stores, and mail-order outlets.

2 SERVINGS

2/3 cup low-fat milk

6 cardamom pods

5 whole cloves

4 black peppercorns

1 (about 1½ inches long) cinnamon stick

¼ teaspoon vanilla extract

1 tea bag

1 cup boiling water

2 to 3 tablespoons granulated sugar

In a saucepan over low heat, combine the milk, cardamom, cloves, peppercorns, cinnamon stick, and vanilla. Simmer for 5 minutes.

Meanwhile, in a mug, combine the tea bag and boiling water. Let steep for 5 minutes.

Remove the milk from the heat and stir in 2 tablespoons of the sugar until dissolved. Remove the tea bag and fill mug with strained hot milk mixture. Taste and add the remaining tablespoon sugar if needed.

PER SERVING

Calories	100
Fat	1 g
Saturated fat	0.5 g
Cholesterol	8 mg
Sodium	40 mg
Carbohydrate	17 g
Dietary fiber	0 g
Sugars	17 g
Protein	3 g
Calcium	100 mg
Potassium	210 mg

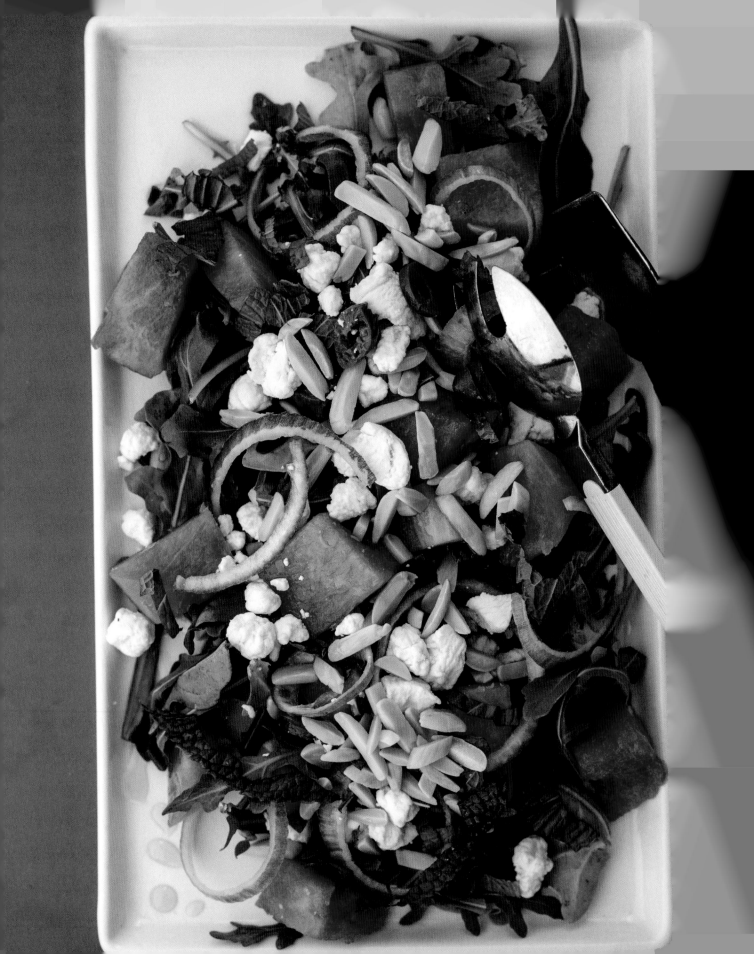

Arugula and Watermelon Salad

This salad tickles your tongue with different flavor profiles. The watermelon is sweet and refreshing, goat cheese and olives add saltiness, and the mint and arugula supply herbal and peppery notes. Slivers of red onion add a touch of pungency.

A honey-lime dressing is the perfect complement, and toasted almonds add crunch.

4 TO 6 SERVINGS

2 tablespoons fresh lime juice

2 tablespoons olive oil

1 tablespoon honey

6 cups arugula

¼ cup slivered fresh mint leaves

2 tablespoons sliced Kalamata olives

1 tablespoon very thinly sliced red onion

3 cups (¾-inch) cubed fresh watermelon, patted dry

⅓ cup crumbled goat cheese

2 tablespoons slivered almonds, toasted

In a bowl, whisk the lime juice, olive oil, and honey. Set aside.

In a bowl, combine the arugula, mint, olives, and red onion and toss to combine. Add half the dressing and toss to lightly coat. Top with the watermelon, goat cheese, and almonds and drizzle with the remaining dressing to taste.

PER SERVING

Calories	180
Fat	12 g
Saturated fat	2.5 g
Cholesterol	10 mg
Sodium	115 mg
Carbohydrate	17 g
Dietary fiber	2 g
Sugars	13 g
Protein	4 g
Calcium	90 mg
Potassium	300 mg

 TIP If you are experiencing neutropenia, omit the goat cheese.

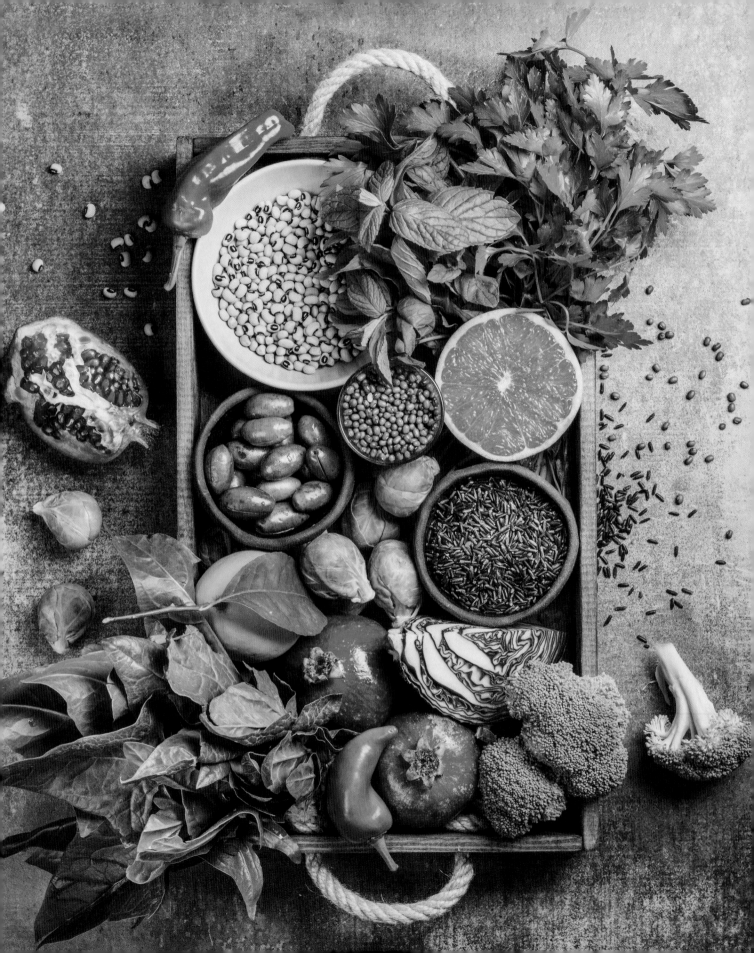

AFTER TREATMENT: EATING WELL, STAYING WELL

Life after cancer treatment will be different for everyone, and each person's nutritional needs will vary as well. You probably want to do whatever you can to stay healthy and keep the cancer from recurring. The biggest challenge may be how to begin to rebuild health following a challenging treatment. Your body will be recovering and healing for some time after treatment ends, and a nutritious diet can help that healing to continue. Your nutritional needs will naturally change over time as you heal and recover.

Although many of the side effects related to cancer and its treatment will go away after treatment ends, there may be some lingering effects that can make eating well more difficult. If you've had surgery or some types of radiation, you may still experience lasting effects—especially if you've had surgery to remove part of your stomach or intestines or have undergone radiation therapy to these areas. People who have received head and neck radiation therapy are at greater risk for dental decay because of treatment-related dry mouth. Those who have received chest radiation may have difficulty swallowing because of treatment-related changes, like narrowing or loss of flexibility of the esophagus.

After treatment ends, you may continue to experience fatigue, taste changes, and changes in bowel and urinary function, and you may still struggle with pain or upset stomach. These treatment-related side effects can affect your appetite and ability to eat. At times, it may be difficult to muster the strength and energy to plan, shop, and cook your meals.

Talk with your registered dietitian (RD) and other members of your health care team about any ongoing challenges you are facing. They can help you set up a nutritional plan that is tailored to your individual situation.

A NEW EATING PLAN: HEALTHFUL EATING FOR LIFE

The ideal wellness plan after treatment will be designed to replenish nutrient stores in your body, rebuild muscle strength, and help manage or correct lingering problems. Eating enough to maintain a healthy weight and being physically active are crucial for a speedy recovery.

A diet containing a variety of healthy protein sources (such as fish and poultry), vegetables, fruits, whole grains, and legumes reduces cancer risk. These foods contain vitamins, minerals, and phytochemicals that help the body fight cancer. This type of diet may also reduce the risk of cancer recurrence and secondary cancers.

TIPS FOR HEALTHY EATING AFTER CANCER

■ Check with your health care team for any continuing food or diet restrictions.

■ Choose a variety of foods from all food groups. Try to eat at least 2½ cups of fruits and vegetables each day, including citrus fruits and dark green and deep yellow vegetables.

■ Eat plenty of high-fiber foods, such as whole grain breads and cereals.

■ Decrease calories in your meals by baking or broiling foods, rather than frying.

■ Limit your intake of red meat (beef, pork, or lamb) to no more than three to four servings a week.

■ Avoid processed, salt-cured, and smoked meats (including bacon, sausage, and deli meats).

■ Choose low-fat or nonfat milk and dairy products.

■ If you choose to drink alcohol, limit the amount to no more than one drink per day for women and two drinks for men. Alcohol is known to increase cancer risk.

HOW TO INCORPORATE MORE FRUITS AND VEGETABLES INTO YOUR DAILY DIET

Many of us do not get the recommended amount of fruits and vegetables each day. As a whole, produce is power-packed with vitamins, minerals, antioxidants, and phytochemicals. Colorful fruits and vegetables tend to have the most antioxidants and phytochemicals, but we don't know which are most protective against cancer, so it's best to try to eat a variety each day.

These are some simple ways to incorporate more produce in your diet:

■ Try hearty meatless meals, such as spinach lasagna, vegetarian chili, or vegetarian pizza, a couple of times a week.

■ Try using vegetables or legumes in the place of meat. These foods are hearty and help to satisfy your hunger. Some easy choices are marinated, roasted portobello mushrooms, baked eggplant with tomatoes and onion, or firm tofu mixed into a stir-fry with brown rice and vegetables.

- Experiment with one new produce item each time you shop for groceries. Try making a mango salsa with onion, cilantro, and red bell pepper; add some julienned jicama to your salad; or bake a spaghetti squash and serve as a side dish.

- Start your day off with fruit. Add apple slices to your oatmeal, toss raisins into your bran cereal, or slice bananas and add to your yogurt.

- Snack on bell pepper strips, baby carrots dipped in hummus, or sliced, fresh fruit and low-fat or nonfat cottage cheese or yogurt.

- Get in the habit of always including a fruit and/or vegetable in every meal and snack, as in these examples:

  - Omelet with broccoli and tomatoes

  - Cereal with berries

  - Pizza with spinach and mushrooms

  - Banana and peanut butter

  - Hummus with carrots, cucumber, or peppers

  - Sandwiches with tomato, lettuce, spinach, or peppers

Look for opportunities to add fruits/vegetables to recipes:

- Add fruit or shredded vegetables to quick breads and muffins (raisins, dried cherries, mashed bananas, or shredded zucchini or carrots).

- Add fruits or vegetables to grain-based dishes, such as quinoa, pilafs, etc.

- Toss beans into soups and salads.

- Double the amount of vegetables in soups.

Keep fruits and vegetables available and accessible:

- Keep cut-up produce in your fridge or washed produce in a bowl on the counter.

- Stash dried fruit in your bag, desk drawer, or glove compartment.

- Take a mini cooler in your car, stocked with fruits or cut-up vegetables for those days you have to leave work early for appointments, to pick up kids, get to sports practices, etc.

- If you buy canned fruits or vegetables, select fruits in 100 percent fruit juice and low- or no-sodium vegetables.

- If you buy frozen or dried fruits or vegetables, select fruits with no added sugar and frozen veggies without added sauces, cheese, or butter.

Use these strategies to prevent produce from going to waste:

- Plan your meals/snacks ahead of time. Don't buy more than you can reasonably use in a week.

- If you shop on the weekend, plan to use "sturdier" vegetables later in the week (for example, use mushrooms and leafy greens early and carrots and broccoli later).

- Store fruits and vegetables separately in different drawers.

- Keep produce in the produce drawer in plastic bags with holes punched in them.

- Cook leftover veggies and freeze to use in omelets or soup when defrosted.

STRIVE TO ACHIEVE A HEALTHY BODY WEIGHT

Cancer treatment may have caused you to gain or lose weight. Talk to your health care team about how to achieve a weight that is healthy for you. Get their support and guidance.

If You Need to Gain Weight

If you need to gain weight, your doctor, nurse, or RD may suggest eating frequently and incorporating high-calorie, high-protein snacks, such as nutritional supplements, milk shakes and smoothies, peanut butter, hummus and vegetables, whole grain bread, and cheese. Gaining weight is not easy for everyone, and it may take time. A weight gain of a pound or two each week is excellent progress.

Even after treatment, large meals may seem overwhelming or unappealing. You may still have a decreased appetite or feel full shortly after you start eating. The following suggestions can help you get the most from your meals:

- Eat small meals or snacks six to eight times a day instead of three main meals.

- Drink hot chocolate, fruit juices, and nectars that are high in calories.

- Keep your favorite snack foods available and around, at home and at work.

- Eat your favorite foods at any time of the day. For example, eat breakfast foods for lunch or dinner, or soups or sandwiches in the morning.

- Include different colors and textures in your meals to make them more appealing.

- Eat your meals in a pleasant setting with family or friends.

- Pleasant smells, such as bread baking or coffee brewing, may help boost your appetite.

If You Need to Lose Weight

Many people want to lose weight following treatment. The best time to tackle weight loss is after treatment, when you've had time to recover. Even then, most health professionals advocate a program of modest weight loss (one to two pounds per week), to be carefully monitored. Talk with your RD or doctor and seek help to set weight-loss goals that are realistic and healthy for your situation.

These foods and cooking methods are good choices to help you stay within a healthful eating plan that is focused on losing weight:

- Raw vegetables with a small amount of low-calorie dip

- Lettuce or spinach salads with vegetables and with dressing on the side

- Steamed vegetables with lemon; vegetables grilled with a spritz of oil

- Lean poultry, sautéed with vegetables

- Seafood that is broiled, baked, steamed, blackened, or poached

- A baked potato topped with broccoli or other sautéed vegetables, or salsa, cilantro, Greek yogurt, and avocado

Eating Out While Trying to Lose Weight

Restaurant meals tend to be higher in calories, fat, sugar, and salt than meals we make at home, so eating out can be difficult when you are trying to lose weight. The good news is that you can eat well away from home. With some nutrition know-how, you don't have to give up on your plans to eat healthy.

The way foods are prepared—and their ingredients—can give you clues as to whether a menu item is a good choice when you are trying to eat better. If you can't tell how a food is prepared or what's in the dish you're considering, ask your server. And don't hesitate to ask for things prepared the way you want them!

Try to look for healthy choices within each course of your meal:

■ Start off with vegetable or seafood appetizers. Avoid anything fried or breaded. Where soups are concerned, broth- or vegetable-based is the best choice. Think gazpacho or lentil soup instead of clam chowder. Avoid breads, such as rolls, croissants, biscuits, or cornbread, which add calories without many nutrients.

■ Vegetables by nature are low in calories and packed with fiber and other disease-fighting nutrients. To keep calories low, choose vegetables seasoned with lemon and/or herbs and spices instead of butter or margarine. If ordering a salad, watch out for toppings that quickly add calories, such as cheese, eggs, and meat. Prepared salads, such as chicken, tuna, egg, pasta, and coleslaw, are frequently made with mayonnaise or other high-calorie salad dressings.

■ For entrées, focus mostly on plant-based foods: vegetables, whole grains, and legumes. Look for seafood or poultry prepared without added fat. Choose dishes flavored with herbs and spices rather than rich cream sauces.

■ It's also a good idea to consider what you're drinking, since beverages can be loaded with calories—a 32-ounce soda has 400 calories! Opt for water, unsweetened iced tea, or sparkling water.

WHAT A NORMAL PORTION LOOKS LIKE

In addition to thinking about what you eat, it's also important to think about how much you're eating. Here's a visual guide to help you get familiar with what a normal portion of food should look like.

FOOD	VISUAL CUE	
1 cup broccoli	Baseball	
Potato	Computer mouse	
Medium apple or orange	Tennis ball	
1/2 cup chopped or cooked fruit	Computer mouse	
1/2 cup brown rice	Computer mouse	
1 cup pasta or dry cereal	Fist (with fingers tucked in)	
2-3 ounces cooked meat, poultry, or fish	Deck of cards	
2 tablespoons peanut butter	Ping pong ball	
1/4 cup dried fruit	Ping pong ball	

Reprinted from The American Cancer Society New Healthy Eating Cookbook. *© Copyright 2016.*

PANTRY STAPLES

Keeping healthy staples on hand can make it easier for you to put nutritious meals or snacks together quickly. This sample pantry staples list can be adapted according to your likes and dislikes.

In the Cupboard

- Dried beans and lentils

- Canned no-salt-added beans, such as black beans, chickpeas, cannellini beans, pinto beans, kidney beans, black-eyed peas, and vegetarian or low-fat refried beans

- Grains, such as brown rice (and instant brown rice), quinoa, wheat berries, bulgur, barley, and farro

- Pastas, including orzo, soba, macaroni, and rice noodles, and whole wheat pastas, such as spaghetti, penne, bowties, and couscous

- Whole wheat crackers, whole grain cereals, and popcorn

- Hot cereals, such as oatmeal (steel-cut, quick-cooking, and rolled)

- Canned tomatoes (diced or whole), salsa, and pasta sauces (watch for added salt and sugar)

- No-sugar-added applesauce and canned fruits in 100 percent juice

- Dried fruits, such as raisins, dates, figs, apricots, prunes, and blueberries (preferably without added sugar)

- Canned tuna or salmon (packed in water)

- Peanut butter and other nut butters

- Nuts, such as almonds, walnuts, and cashews

- Vinegars, such as balsamic, rice, red wine, and apple cider

- Oils, including olive oil, canola oil, and nonstick cooking spray

In the Refrigerator

- Fresh vegetables and fruits
- Nonfat yogurts (without added sugar)
- Reduced-fat or regular cheeses
- Corn or whole wheat tortillas
- Eggs
- Minced garlic
- Hummus

In the Freezer

- Frozen vegetables, such as spinach, broccoli, edamame, peas, corn, and mixed vegetables (without added butter or sauces)
- Frozen fruits, such as berries and peaches (without added sugar)
- Chicken breasts and ground turkey breast
- Fish, such as salmon, flounder, tilapia, and red snapper

STAYING ACTIVE

Staying active must be part of any healthy lifestyle plan. Talk with your doctor first, and start slowly, gradually increasing the amount of exercise you do, especially if you were not active before treatment. Exercise can help you regain strength and flexibility, maintain an optimal weight, reduce stress, strengthen the immune system, and even relieve symptoms such as depression, anxiety, or irregular bowel movements. Regular exercise can also reintroduce a sense of autonomy that is sometimes lost during treatment.

A well-rounded activity plan includes aerobic exercise, strength training, and flexibility exercises. Even when performed in small but regular increments, this balanced approach to physical activity provides real benefits for the body. As a goal, the American Cancer Society recommends at least thirty minutes of activity on five or more days of the week, including strength training exercises at least two days per week.

FINDING HELP WITH PHYSICAL ACTIVITY AFTER CANCER TREATMENT

Certified Trainer in Cancer Exercise: To find a certified trainer, contact the American College of Sports Medicine at www.acsm.org or (317) 637-9200.

LiveStrong at the YMCA: To find a program in your area, contact the YMCA in your community.

Cancer Rehabilitation Experts: Physical therapists are available within your local or community health system. Ask your doctor for a referral.

It can understandably be difficult sometimes for cancer survivors to get moving. Fatigue, lack of interest, sedentary lifestyle prior to the cancer diagnosis, body image issues, and lingering effects from treatment are all possible barriers. But there are many simple ways to be more active and gradually incorporate more activity into your life:

- Use stairs rather than an elevator or escalator.

- If you can, walk or bike to your destination.

- Exercise at lunch with your workmates, family, or friends.

- Take a 10-minute exercise break at work to stretch or take a quick walk.

- Walk to visit coworkers rather than sending e-mails or calling.

- Go dancing with your spouse or friends.

- Plan active vacations rather than driving-only trips.

- Wear a pedometer every day and watch your daily steps increase. Try to work up to 10,000 steps per day.

- Park far from a store and walk.

- Join a sports team or take up dance or zumba.

- Plan for gradual increases in the length and frequency of exercise sessions.

Start slowly and be patient with yourself. The ultimate goal is to incorporate more physical activity as a permanent part of your life as part of better health after treatment.

BIBLIOGRAPHY

Eating well during and after your cancer treatment. Memorial Sloan Kettering Cancer Center website. https://www.mskcc.org/pdf/cancer-care/patient-education/eating-well-during-and-after-your-treatment?mode=large. Posted February 16, 2018. Accessed February 21, 2018.

Espat, Adelina. Does sugar cause cancer? MD Anderson Cancer Center website. https://www.mdanderson.org/publications/focused-on-health/may-2015/FOH-cancer-love-sugar.html. Published May 2015. Accessed February 21, 2018.

Food safety guidelines. Seattle Cancer Care Alliance website. https://www.seattlecca.org/nutrition/food-safety-guidelines. Accessed February 21, 2018.

General oncology diet guidelines. Seattle Cancer Care Alliance website. https://www.seattlecca.org/food-and-safety-general-oncology-diet-guidelines. Accessed February 21, 2018.

Grant B, Hamilton K, Thomson C, Bloch A. *American Cancer Society Complete Guide to Nutrition for Cancer Survivors.* Atlanta, GA: American Cancer Society; 2010.

Iron in your diet. Memorial Sloan Kettering Cancer Center website. https://www.mskcc.org/cancer-care/patient-education/iron-your-diet. Updated August 7, 2015. Accessed February 20, 2018.

Janis M. Iron deficiency anemia in cancer patients. *Oncology & Hematology Review.* 2012;8(2):74–80. DOI: 10.17925/OHR.2012.08.2.74.

Kushi LH, Doyle C, McCullough M, Rock CL, Demark-Wahnefried,W, Bandera EV, Gapstur S, Patel AV, Andrews K, Gansler T, and The American Cancer Society 2010 Nutrition and Physical Activity Guidelines Advisory Committee (2012), American Cancer Society guidelines on nutrition and physical activity for cancer prevention. *CA: A Cancer Journal for Clinicians.* 2012;62:30–67. doi: 10.3322/caac.20140.

National Cancer Institute. Eating hints: Before, during, and after cancer treatment. NIH Publication No. 18-7157. https://www.cancer.gov/publications/patient-education/eatinghints.pdf. Published January 2018. Accessed February 21, 2018.

National Institutes of Health, Office of Dietary Supplements. Magnesium fact sheet for health professionals. https://ods.od.nih.gov/factsheets/Magnesium-HealthProfessional/. Updated February 11, 2016. Accessed February 21, 2018.

Nutrition after treatment ends. American Cancer Society website. https://www.cancer.org/treatment/survivorship-during-and-after-treatment/staying-active/nutrition/nutrition-during-treatment/after-treatment-ends.html. Updated July 15, 2015. Accessed February 21, 2018.

Nutrition and physical activity during and after cancer treatment: Answers to common questions. American Cancer Society website. https://www.cancer.org/treatment/survivorship-during-and-after-treatment/staying-active/nutrition/nutrition-and-physical-activity-during-and-after-cancer-treatment.html. Updated April 11, 2013. Accessed February 21, 2018.

Potassium in diet. MedlinePlus website. https://medlineplus.gov/ency/article/002413.htm. Updated April 24, 2016. Accessed February 21, 2018.

Rock CL, Doyle C, Demark-Wahnefried W, Meyerhardt J, Courneya KS, Schwartz AL, Bandera EV, Hamilton KK, Grant B, McCullough M, Byers T, Gansler T. Nutrition and physical activity guidelines for cancer survivors. *CA Cancer J Clin.* 2012;62:242–274.

Salmon, Maureen. 8 Tips for Managing Weight During and After Cancer Treatment. Memorial Sloan Kettering Cancer Center website. https://www.mskcc.org/blog/8-tips-managing-weight-during-and-after-treatment. Published June 26, 2015. Accessed June 26, 2018.

Seattle Cancer Care Alliance and Fred Hutchinson Cancer Research Center. Adult and pediatric guidelines for the use of herbal and nutrient supplements during hematopoietic stem cell transplantation (HSCT) and high-dose chemotherapy. Fred Hutchinson Cancer Research Center website. https://www.fredhutch.org/content/dam/public/Treatment-Suport/Long-Term-Follow-Up/herbal_sup_2510_0.pdf. Accessed February 21, 2018.

US Food and Drug Administration. Food safety for people with cancer. https://www.fda.gov/downloads/Food/FoodborneIllnessContaminants/UCM312761.pdf. Published September 2006. Updated September 2011. Accessed February 21, 2018.

US Food and Drug Administration. Guidance for industry: A food labeling guide (16. Appendix H: Rounding the values according to FDA rounding rules). http://www.fda.gov/Food/GuidanceRegulation/GuidanceDocumentsRegulatoryInformation/LabelingNutrition/ucm064932.htm. Revised June 24, 2015. Accessed April 27, 2016.

White, Nicole. Weight Gain Can Be an Unexpected Side Effect of Cancer Treatment. City of Hope website. https://www.cityofhope.org/blog/weight-gain-and-cancer. Published February 18, 2014. Accessed June 25, 2018.

RECIPES BY SIDE EFFECT

N RECIPES FOR NAUSEA

Carrot-Ginger Drink (page 34)

Skillet Chicken with Root Vegetables (page 36)

Quinoa-Sweet Potato Patties (page 37)

Spring Minestrone (page 39)

Chicken Broth Two Ways (page 40)

Egg Roll-Up with Parsley and Dill (page 42)

Mini Muffin Tin Chicken-Ricotta Meatballs (page 44)

Pineapple-Mango Slushies (page 45)

Steamed Chicken with Vegetables and Rice (page 47)

Pumpkin-Ginger Mini Muffins (page 48)

One-Bowl Gluten-Free Banana Pancakes (page 49)

Miso-Chicken Soup (page 50)

Ginger-Lime Spritzer (page 52)

Blueberry-Corn Mini Muffins (page 53)

Lemon-Ginger Biscotti (page 54)

Mushroom Broth (page 56)

On-the-Go Snack Mix (page 57)

Strawberry-Watermelon-Mint Cooler (page 59)

Chicken Noodle Soup (page 60)

Chicken Congee (page 68)

Rehydration Drinks (page 70)

Vegetable Broth (page 74)

Baked Rice Balls (page 75)

Lemon-Herb Tilapia Packets (page 76)

Oatmeal-Banana-Peach Smoothie (page 78)

Brown Sugar-Oatmeal Muffins (page 79)

Fruited Gelatin (page 82)

Cran-Apple Slushie (page 83)

Lemon Rice (page 87)

Mashed Potato-Chicken Patties (page 91)

Herb-Flecked Popovers (page 93)

Egg Drop Soup (page 136)

Golden Milk (page 139)

Cranberry-Lime Granita (page 148)

Fruity Yogurt Bark (page 177)

Strawberry-Blueberry "Mocktail" (page 228)

D RECIPES FOR DIARRHEA

Spring Minestrone (page 39)

Chicken Broth Two Ways (page 40)

Egg Roll-Up with Parsley and Dill (page 42)

Mini Muffin Tin Chicken-Ricotta Meatballs (page 44)

Steamed Chicken with Vegetables and Rice (page 47)

One-Bowl Gluten-Free Banana Pancakes (page 49)

Ginger-Lime Spritzer (page 52)

Lemon-Ginger Biscotti (page 54)

Mushroom Broth (page 56)

Strawberry-Watermelon-Mint Cooler (page 59)

Chicken Noodle Soup (page 60)

Miso-Glazed Salmon (page 67)

Chicken Congee (page 68)

Rehydration Drinks (page 70)

Fish In "Tomato Water" (page 73)

Vegetable Broth (page 74)

Baked Rice Balls (page 75)

Lemon-Herb Tilapia Packets (page 76)

Oatmeal-Banana-Peach Smoothie (page 78)

Brown Sugar-Oatmeal Muffins (page 79)

c RECIPES FOR CONSTIPATION

TS RECIPES FOR TROUBLE SWALLOWING

SM RECIPES FOR SORE MOUTH OR THROAT

WL RECIPES FOR UNINTENTIONAL WEIGHT LOSS

TC RECIPES FOR TASTE CHANGES

METRIC EQUIVALENTS

VOLUME

(ml=milliliter)

¼ teaspoon	1 ml
½ teaspoon	2.5 ml
¾ teaspoon	4 ml
1 teaspoon	5 ml
1 ¼ teaspoons	6 ml
1 ½ teaspoons	7.5 ml
1 ¾ teaspoons	8.5 ml
2 teaspoons	10 ml
1 tablespoon	15 ml
2 tablespoons	30 ml
¼ cup	59 ml
⅓ cup	79 ml
½ cup	118 ml
⅔ cup	158 ml
¾ cup	178 ml
1 cup	237 ml
1 ½ cups	355 ml
2 cups (1 pint)	473 ml
3 cups	710 ml
4 cups (1 quart)	.95 liter
1.06 quarts	1 liter
4 quarts (1 gallon)	3.8 liters

WEIGHT

0.35 ounce	1 gram
¼ ounce	7 grams
½ ounce	14 grams
¾ ounce	21 grams
1 ounce	28 grams
1 ½ ounces	42.5 grams
2 ounces	57 grams
3 ounces	85 grams
4 ounces	113 grams
5 ounces	142 grams
6 ounces	170 grams
7 ounces	198 grams
8 ounces	227 grams
16 ounces (1 pound)	454 grams
2.2 pounds	1 kilogram

INDEX